HYPERTROPHIC CARDIOMYOPATHY:

For Patients, Their Families, and Interested Physicians

By

Barry J. Maron, M.D.
Minneapolis Heart Institute Foundation
Minneapolis, Minnesota

With Lisa Salberg
of
The Hypertrophic Cardiomyopathy Association (HCMA)

For the use and benefit of patients afflicted with this disorder, their families, and treating physicians, and with a commitment to the dissemination of information regarding this uncommon, complex and often misunderstood disease.

Futura Media Services, Inc.
Armonk, NY

Library of Congress Cataloging-in-Publication Data
Maron, Barry J.,
    Hypertrophic cardiomyopathy: for patients, their families and interested physicians / Barry J. Maron -- .
       p. ; cm.
    ISBN 0-913848-05-0 (alk. paper)
    1. I. Title.
    [DNLM:]

                                                    2001018758

Published by
Futura Media Services, Inc.
135 Bedford Road
Armonk, New York 10504
www.futuraco.com

LC#: 2001018758
ISBN#: 0-913848-05-0

Printed in part with a grant from the Medtronic Foundation.

Every effort has been made to ensure that the information in this book is as up to date and accurate as possible at the time of publication. However, due to the constant developments in medicine, neither the author, nor the editor, nor the publisher can accept any legal or any other responsibility for any errors or omissions that may occur.

Printed in the United States of America.

This book is printed on acid-free paper.

Acknowledgements

I wish to acknowledge the constant and ongoing support, for more than 30 years, which made this book possible—from my wife Donna and my two children, Marty (who is a physician) and Bradley (who will be so, shortly), as well as our new daughter-in-law, Dr. Jill Maron. Also, the substantial contribution of Terri Hanson in the extensive preparation of the manuscript is greatly appreciated.

Barry J. Maron, M.D.
Minneapolis, Minnesota

Cover: For an explanation of the cover illustrations, see pages 10–12.

Dedication

This book is dedicated to the memory of Lori Anne Flanigan, who passed away June 15, 1995 of hypertrophic cardiomyopathy, at the age of only 36 years. Lori is remembered as a wonderful mother, sister, daughter, and friend. The Hypertrophic Cardiomyopathy Association was founded in her memory.

In addition, many thanks to Carolyn Biro, Fred Kanter, Dan Kanter, and the entire Flanigan/Salberg family for their friendship and support.

We also wish to thank the Medtronic Foundation for their interest in hypertrophic cardiomyopathy, and for their support in making this book possible.

Contents

Introduction

This handbook is designed for those interested in learning more about the heart condition, hypertrophic cardiomyopathy (HCM). It has been created through the collaboration of expert physicians, other medical personnel, and patients with the condition, and seeks to address the major questions and concerns of patients and their families regarding HCM. We also believe this book will be useful to physicians (including cardiologists) in developing an understanding of HCM. While the language of the text was designed largely with nonmedically oriented individuals in mind (medical terminology and jargon is kept to a minimum and very basic anatomy and physiology is discussed), this should not discourage medical personnel at any level from using and benefiting from the information included in this book.

This volume, therefore, is not only intended to provide a basic review of a complex condition, but rather is a scientific treatise written and organized in such a way as to be appropriate and accessible to as wide an audience as possible, including patients without medical or scientific background. The clinical concepts presented here concerning HCM can be regarded as relevant, important, and up-to-date, regardless of the precise language used to express these perspectives.

What Is Hypertrophic Cardiomyopathy?

Cardiomyopathy is a general term describing any condition in which the heart muscle is structurally and functionally abnormal (the heart itself is a specialized type of muscle). There are four basic types of cardiomyopathy: **hypertrophic, dilated, restrictive,** and **arrhythmogenic right ventricular cardiomyopathy**. This volume will focus only on the first type, *hypertrophic cardiomyopathy (HCM)*.

Basically, HCM is a genetic disease affecting the heart muscle. The most consistent feature of HCM is excessive thickening of the wall of the heart muscle (*hypertrophy* = heart muscle thickening; *cardiomyopathy* = diseased heart muscle). The consequences of HCM to patients are related, in part or solely, to the abnormally thickened heart muscle, which in turn is a consequence of the basic genetic defect. Hypertrophy may be widespread throughout the left ventricle, though not necessarily, and there is no single "typical" pattern of muscle thickening.

1

The heart (specifically the left ventricle) may also thicken in other individuals who do not have HCM, either as a result of high blood pressure, obstructive heart valve disease, or even prolonged and intense athletic training in certain sports. The type of hypertrophy associated with high blood pressure is often referred to as "secondary" (i.e., a secondary consequence of the increased blood pressure). In HCM, however, the muscular thickening of the heart wall is primary, i.e., due to a genetic defect and not a reaction to other factors. In addition, when the heart muscle of HCM is viewed under a light microscope, it usually shows several particular abnormalities, the most prominent of which is called *myocardial cell (myocyte) disarray or disorganization* (Figure 1), in which normal parallel alignment of heart muscle cells has been lost and many of the muscle cells are arranged in a characteristically chaotic and disorganized pattern. It is likely that this cell disarray interferes with normal electrical transmission of impulses and predisposes some patients to irregularities of heart rhythm, as well as altering the heart contraction.

Historical Perspective and Names

The first modern description of HCM was in 1958 by a British pathologist, Dr. Donald Teare, who likened the disease to a tumor of the heart. Since then, many different terms have been used to refer to this condition, and this issue of nomenclature *is* confusing (Figure 2).

Remarkably, HCM has been given over 75 different names by individual clinicians and scientists over the last 40 years. No other disease has been described by so many varying terms. Why has this occurred? The principal reason for the proliferation of names undoubtedly has been the heterogeneity and diversity with which the condition is expressed, a major point in understanding HCM. Since very few cardiologists have treated large numbers of patients with HCM, they have often come to regard the overall disease based only on their personal (and sometimes limited) experiences.

Many of the alternate names for HCM are misleading since they emphasize obstruction to left ventricular outflow which is a highly visible feature of the disease but, in fact, is probably present under resting conditions in no more than about 20-25% of all patients. Therefore, names for this disease have included *idiopathic hypertrophic subaortic stenosis (IHSS)*, which was the first popular term used in the U.S.; "stenosis" means obstruction. The same can be said for *hypertrophic obstructive cardiomyopathy (HOCM)* which is still a widely used term in the United Kingdom.

Normal Cell Structure

Myocardial Disarray

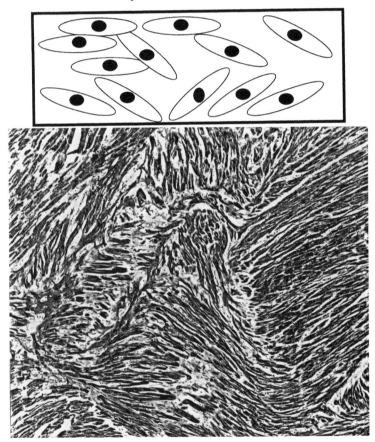

Figure 1. *The cell structure and architecture of the HCM heart.* Diagrams contrast the regular and parallel alignment of muscle cells in the normal heart (**top**) with the irregular, disorganized alignment of cells (myocardial disarray) found in some areas of the HCM heart (**middle**). A picture of an actual area of an HCM heart (from a histologic section) (**bottom**) shows a disorganized chaotic arrangement of cardiac muscle cells (myocytes).

TERMS USED TO DESCRIBE HYPERTROPHIC CARDIOMYOPATHY

Acquired aortic subvalvular stenosis
Apical asymmetric septal hypertrophy
Apical hypertrophic cardiomyopathy
Apical hypertrophic nonobstructive
  cardiomyopathy
Apical hypertrophy
Asymmetric left ventricular hypertrophy
Asymmetric septal hypertrophy
Asymmetrical apical hypertrophy
Asymmetrical hypertrophic cardiomyopathy
Asymmetrical hypertrophy of the heart
Brock's disease
Diffuse muscular subaortic stenosis
Diffuse subvalvular aortic stenosis
Dynamic hypertrophic subaortic stenosis
Dynamic muscular subaortic stenosis
Familial hypertrophic subaortic stenosis
Familial muscular subaortic stenosis
Familial myocardial disease
Functional aortic stenosis
Functional aortic subvalvar stenosis
Functional hypertrophic subaortic stenosis
Functional obstructive cardiomyopathy
Functional obstruction of the left ventricle
Functional obstructive subvalvular
  aortic stenosis
Functional subaortic stenosis
Hereditary cardiovascular dysplasia
Hypertrophic apical cardiomyopathy
HYPERTROPHIC CARDIOMYOPATHY
Hypertrophic constrictive cardiomyopathy
Hypertrophic disease
Hypertrophic hyperkinetic cardiomyopathy
Hypertrophic infundibular aortic stenosis
Hypertrophic nonobstructive apical
  cardiomyopathy
Hypertrophic nonobstructive cardiomyopathy
Hypertrophic nonobstructive cardiomyopathy
  with giant negative T waves
Hypertrophic obstructive cardiomyopathy
Hypertrophic obstructive cardiomyopathy
  of left ventricle
Hypertrophic restrictive cardiomyopathy
Hypertrophic stenosing cardiomyopathy

Hypertrophic subaortic stenosis
Idiopathic hypertrophic cardiomyopathy
Idiopathic hypertrophic obstructive cardiomyopathy
Idiopathic hypertrophic subaortic stenosis
Idiopathic hypertrophic subvalvular stenosis
Idiopathic muscular hypertrophic subaortic stenosis
Idiopathic muscular stenosis of the left ventricle
Idiopathic myocardial hypertrophy
Idiopathic ventricular septal hypertrophy
Irregular hypertrophic cardiomyopathy
Left ventricular muscular stenosis
Low subvalvular aortic stenosis
Mid-ventricular hypertrophic cardiomyopathy
Mid-ventricular hypertrophic obstructive
  cardiomyopathy
Mid-ventricular obstruction
Muscular aortic stenosis
Muscular hypertrophic stenosis of the left ventricle
Muscular stenosis of the left ventricle
Muscular subaortic stenosis
Muscular subvalvular aortic stenosis
Non-dilated cardiomyopathy
Nonobstructive hypertrophic cardiomyopathy
Obstructive cardiomyopathy
Obstructive hypertrophic aortic stenosis
Obstructive hypertrophic cardiomyopathy
Obstructive hypertrophic myocardiopathy
Obstructive myocardiopathy
Pseudoaortic stenosis
Stenosing hypertrophy of the left ventricle
Stenosis of the ejection chamber of left ventricle
Subaortic hypertrophic obstructive cardiomyopathy
Subaortic hypertrophic stenosis
Subaortic idiopathic stenosis
Subaortic muscular stenosis
Subvalvular aortic stenosis
Subvalvular aortic stenosis of the muscular type
Teare's disease
Typical hypertrophic obstructive cardiomyopathy

Figure 2. Many terms (about 75) have been used to refer to HCM over a 4-decade period, which perhaps reflects the diversity with which the disease is expressed.

Presently, virtually all HCM experts and other cardiovascular specialists now regard *hypertrophic cardiomyopathy* as the best single term for the broad disease spectrum. This term emphasizes the *hypertrophy* which is the diagnostic marker in most patients, and the fact that this disease is a *cardiomyopathy* – or heart muscle disorder – without mentioning obstruction (which is present only in a minority of patients). Therefore, the terms "HCM *with* obstruction" or "HCM *without* obstruction" are preferred.

How Common Is HCM?

Recent studies in the U.S. suggest that HCM is more common than was previously believed. It is now estimated that somewhere between about 1 in 500 to 1 in 1000 individuals within the general population have the disease. These figures relate to adults in whom the disease is recognized by echocardiography; many children and other adults could carry a mutant gene for HCM and be completely unaware of that fact. HCM appears to occur throughout the world with most of the scientific interest and reports coming from North America (U.S. and Canada), Japan, and Europe (United Kingdom, Italy, France, Germany, and Switzerland), although reports have also come from South America, Israel, and Australia/New Zealand. HCM appears to be remarkably similar with regard to presentation, heart structure, and prognosis in patients from these diverse areas of the world. One relatively minor exception is the Japanese version of HCM where the apical form of the disease (with wall thickening localized to the tip of the left ventricle) seems to be more common than in other countries – a difference that may be due to unique racial and environmental factors.

What Is the Cause of HCM?

It is important to emphasize that HCM is usually a familial condition and represents a genetically transmitted disease. The pattern of inheritance for HCM is known as ***autosomal dominant***, which means that the disease (and the mutant gene) appears in about 50% of the members in each subsequent generation, and therefore the likelihood of an affected parent transmitting the abnormal gene to their child is statistically about 1 in 2 (Figure 3). However, autosomal dominant inheritance does not necessarily mean that if there are 4 offspring, 2 must be affected – only that this is the statistical probability. In reality, it could be zero of 4 or even 4 of 4 offspring who will carry the mutant gene. Some individuals with this disease appear to be "sporadic" cases – i.e., there are no other relatives in the family who are known to have HCM.

Genetic "skipping" of a generation is rare but can appear to occur when an individual who is a gene carrier does not even have evidence of the disease on the echocardiogram. In such a circumstance, the mutant gene does not actually "skip" a generation – in reality, the HCM gene in that individual simply does not express itself fully, in such a way that we can see evidence of the disease with the echocardiogram (or electrocardiogram).

GENERATIONS

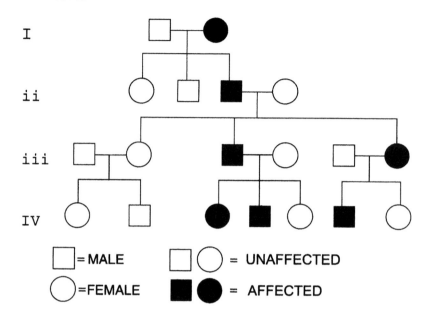

Figure 3. *Family tree.* Shown here are four generations of a family affected by HCM. There is typical *autosomal dominant inheritance* in which the condition is transmitted from one generation to another. Each offspring of an affected person has about a 50% chance of inheriting the gene and disease.

At present, a multitude of mutations in 9 genes, which are necessary for the development and contraction of heart muscle cells (in units called **sarcomeres**), have been mapped to their respective chromosomes and isolated from members of families with HCM (some of these mutant genes also exist in skeletal muscle, as well as heart muscle). The 9 genes presently regarded as causing HCM are known in scientific terms as: (1) beta-myosin heavy chain; (2) cardiac myosin-binding protein C; (3) cardiac troponin T; (4) troponin I; (5) alpha-tropomyosin; (6 and 7) essential and regulatory myosin light chains; (8) actin; and (9) titin. In most patients, HCM is caused by the initial 3 genes on this list, while the other 6 genes each account for only a small fraction of the patients. Additional genes and mutations responsible for HCM will undoubtedly be identified in the future.

A **mutation** is a defect in the DNA code, the protein structure of the gene. These DNA abnormalities may take many forms, but some can be likened to a "spelling error" in the genetic code of DNA such as displacement in the order or sequence of just one of many amino acids (the individual "building blocks" of the gene protein). Indeed, it is striking, and perhaps surprising, that seemingly minor-appearing abnormalities in the gene sequence can make such a profound difference in the structure of the heart, as occurs in HCM.

Patients often inquire about the cause of their mutation, particularly if the gene abnormality has appeared for the first time in a family. This is known as a "de novo" mutation. An example of this would be a newly diagnosed child with HCM, of two parents, each of whom have a normal echocardiogram and no evidence of HCM. Keep in mind that the genetic predisposition to HCM (i.e., the mutant gene) does not always trace back many generations in the same family, but may occur spontaneously and for the first time in a member of the most recent generation. Unfortunately, at present, the environmental factors that do trigger HCM mutations are not known.

The discovery of these gene abnormalities is a major step toward understanding the basic cause of HCM. Ultimately, this may allow laboratory DNA diagnosis from a blood test (or from saliva or a skin smear from inside the mouth) in individual patients. The availability of such a test would be particularly useful for identification of HCM in young children and adolescents, and in any situation where the HCM diagnosis is ambiguous –such as in the case of some athletes in whom it is difficult to distinguish HCM from the effects on the heart of chronic exercise and training. At the present time, however, it is not feasible or practical to obtain such testing for individual patients on a routine basis. This technology remains arduous, time-intensive, and firmly entrenched in the research arena.

Ongoing and future investigations will also focus on the identification of new genes that cause HCM and, ultimately, an understanding of how these genetic abnormalities result in this form of heart disease. There continues to be an effort to distinguish "good" from "bad" HCM genes, which may ultimately prove to be of major value in determining which patients are at high risk for sudden death. For example, at this early stage, some researchers have suggested that generally unfavorable mutations include all those of the troponin T gene and some of beta-myosin heavy chain, while more favorable mutations include those of the myosin-binding protein C gene. At the present time, however, this information is incomplete and it is not possible to make routine definitive assessments on single blood samples. When it becomes possible to identify mutations responsible for HCM rapidly and automatically through advances in "chip technology," we will then be able to make this genetic information more clinically relevant to individual patients.

At present, molecular biologists with a focus on HCM believe that knowledge of the basic genetic defect in individual families will ultimately unlock most of the important secrets of prognosis in this disease, and thereby permit more targeted, definitive, and earlier intervention.

However, such a level of understanding may be many years off, and until that time we must treat patients with available and practical strategies (some of which are powerful and efficacious), which may seem somewhat empirical compared with genetically based interventions.

How Does HCM Alter the Heart?

The Normal Heart (Figures 4 and 5)

First, it is helpful to be familiar with the structure and function of the normal heart in order to understand the abnormalities in HCM. A normal heart has 4 heart chambers (left and right ventricles as the lower chambers; left and right atria as the upper chambers) and 4 valves (mitral and tricuspid; aortic and pulmonary). The walls of the heart are composed of heart muscle cells, as well as collagen and small veins and arteries (called venules and arterioles, respectively). The left ventricular wall is normally about 3 times thicker than the wall of the right ventricle. The left ventricular wall is usually of similar thickness in all areas and, in adults, it measures 12 millimeters (mm) or less on the echocardiogram (in the relaxation phase, diastole). The normal course of blood flow through the heart is shown in Figure 4.

Every normal heartbeat results from an electrical signal starting in the right atrium (sinoatrial node) and passing down through the conducting system of the heart and into the ventricles. The contraction of the heart follows the same sequence.

The Heart in HCM (Figure 5)

In HCM, the left ventricular wall is abnormal by virtue of excessive thickening, while the cavity of the left ventricle is of normal or small size (Figure 5). HCM has often been referred to as an "enlarged heart," but is probably more accurately regarded as "thickened" or "muscular." The distribution of this muscle thickening (or hypertrophy) may take many forms and differ greatly among patients (even those who are related). The particular pattern, precise site, or degree of hypertrophy may vary considerably among patients, which, while not always significant, may be important in selected patients, including those with particularly severe thickening of the left ventricular wall. The most common structural form of HCM involves the muscle thickening located predom-

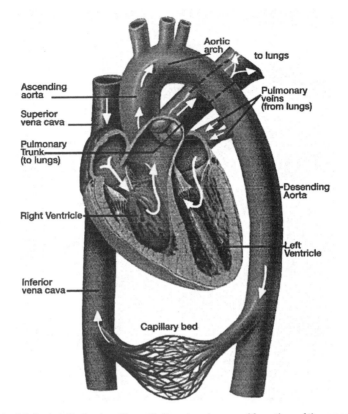

Figure 4. It is helpful to be familiar with the structure and function of the normal heart in order to understand the abnormalities in HCM. This drawing shows a normal heart with heart chambers, valves, and the direction of blood flow. The walls of the heart are composed of specialized muscle known as the *myocardium*. This part of the heart is abnormal in HCM. The arrows show the direction of blood flow through the heart. The right atrium receives unoxygenated blood from the body and transfers it to the right ventricle, which pumps it into the lungs to receive oxygen. Blood returns to the heart from the lungs into the left atrium and is transferred to the left ventricle, which pumps it into the systemic circulation and another cycle.

inantly in the *ventricular septum* – the portion of left ventricular wall that divides the right and left chambers of the heart.

In addition, the absolute thickness of the wall may also vary greatly among patients. On the one hand, HCM may reach thicknesses that far exceed any other cardiac disease – up to 5 times normal. The upper limit of normal wall thickness is 10–12 mm; remarkably, some patients may have thicknesses as much as 40–60 mm (Figure 7). Patients are often very focused on their exact "number" for wall thickness but, in most patients, this precise value is usually of little significance. One exception would be those with extremely thick walls of more than 30

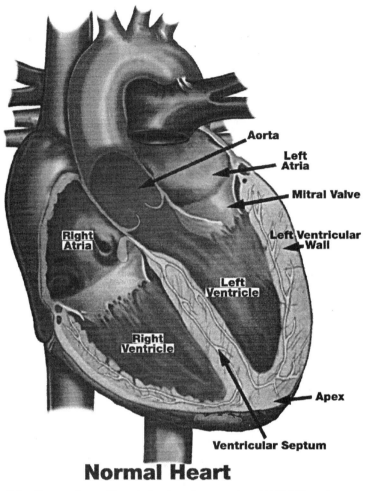

Normal Heart

Figure 5A. *Comparison of heart structure in normal and HCM.* Note that compared to normal (**A**), the HCM heart (**B** and **C**) usually shows thickening of the ventricular septum that is greater than other parts of the left ventricular (LV) wall, whether or not there is obstruction. However, the exact pattern of hypertrophy in HCM can be quite diverse and is not limited to that shown here. The mechanism by which obstruction occurs when the mitral valve comes forward and contacts the septum (arrow), i.e., systolic anterior motion of the mitral valve or SAM, is shown in **C**. *(continued)*

mm or 35 mm, with which increased risk for sudden death has been associated. In contrast, many patients have only mildly increased thickness that may be confined to only a small portion of the wall.

Usually, the hypertrophy in HCM is described as ***asymmetric***, which means that some parts of the wall are thicker than others (Figure 5). It is usually the septum that is thickest, and portions of the left

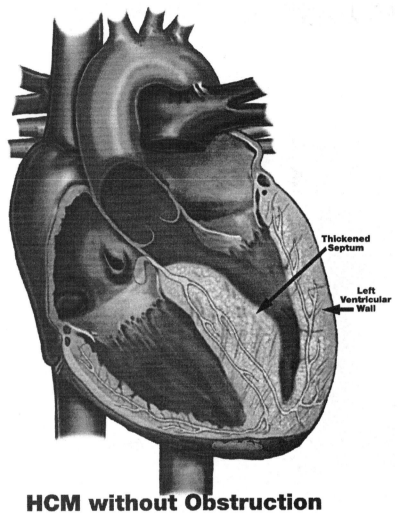

HCM without Obstruction

Figure 5B. *(continued)*

ventricular free wall (i.e., those not part of the septum) that are thinner. The term "*concentric*" means that all portions of the wall are of about the same thickness; this form of hypertrophy is uncommon and, when strictly defined, is present in only about 2% of HCM patients (although it is possibly more common in certain specific patient groups, such as the elderly). Also, in a small proportion of patients (approximately 2%), wall thickening is predominantly at the tip, or *apex,* of the heart. This form of HCM seems to be more common in Japan, and always occurs without obstruction.

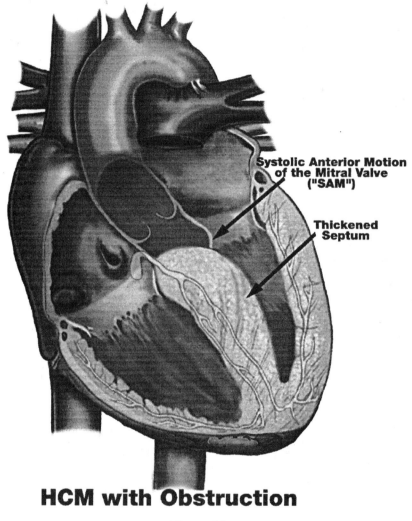

Systolic Anterior Motion of the Mitral Valve ("SAM")

Thickened Septum

HCM with Obstruction

Figure 5C.

HCM is a complex disease, which is well illustrated by the fact that a few adult individuals may harbor a mutant gene for HCM, but nevertheless have normal echocardiograms and electrocardiograms, and therefore completely escape clinical detection. Indeed, such a circumstance is an example of *HCM without hypertrophy*. Based on the available information, however, there does not seem to be significant risk associated with this form of HCM (except in a few selected families), although some of these individuals may "convert" to a more typical appearance of HCM in mid-life by developing a thick heart wall.

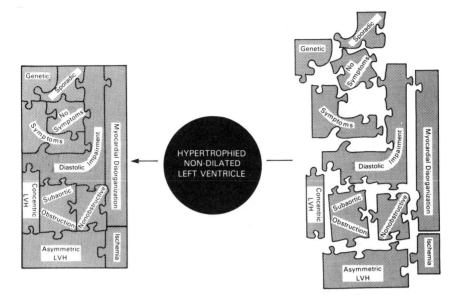

Figure 6. The clinical definition of HCM is based on the presence of left ventricular hypertrophy without cavity enlargement, in a patient who does not have another cardiac (or systemic) disease that itself could potentially produce the particular degree of hypertrophy. This is the criterion for diagnosis that brings together the diverse "jigsaw puzzle" that HCM often appears to be.

Also, other very different heart conditions may mimic HCM by virtue of showing a thick heart, and the distinction may be difficult at times. These include diseases that infiltrate the heart (and other organs), such as amyloidosis, which occurs almost exclusively in older patients, other genetic conditions such as Noonan's syndrome in infants and young children and Fabry's disease in adults, and also some uncommon examples of athlete's heart in which the thickening of the wall is "innocent" (or, benign) and due solely to intense training.

Muscle thickening involving the upper portion of septum is sometimes associated with a unique motion pattern of the mitral valve (Figure 5). In such cases, during the ejection of the blood from the heart (in systole), the mitral valve moves forward and contacts the septum (there should normally be a considerable gap between these two structures) and partially obstructs the outflow of blood from the left side of the heart into the aorta, creating a *pressure gradient* between the aorta and left ventricle. Therefore, ***outflow obstruction*** in HCM is actually caused by mitral valve motion and is not, per se, due to the thickened septum (Figure 5). This is known as ***systolic anterior motion of the mitral valve (SAM).*** The turbulent blood flow produced by obstruction creates a ***murmur*** – a sound that is audible with a stethoscope. Also,

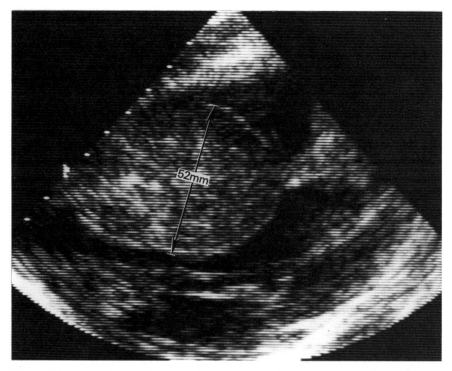

Figure 7. A stop-frame photograph from a two-dimensional echocardiogram of an HCM heart with extreme left ventricular wall thickening. Note that the ventricular septum measures 52 millimeters (mm) in thickness, which is about 5 times normal.

the abnormal motion assumed by the mitral valve may cause blood to leak backward into the left atrium. This leakage is called *mitral regurgitation*. While the thickening of the left ventricular wall is, in fact, the primary abnormality in HCM, the mitral valve may also be enlarged and elongated.

Outflow obstruction, although present in the resting state in only about 20-25% of HCM patients, may account for symptoms such as shortness of breath, fatigue, chest pain, and fainting. The descriptive term, *obstruction,* often has a strong connotation to patients that often may not be entirely deserved. This word refers to only *partial* obstruction (or impedance) to the flow of blood from left ventricle to aorta. Obstruction is not necessarily unfavorable to patients and can be tolerated for many years with no or few symptoms or difficulty. On the other hand, in some patients, severely limiting symptoms can be attributed directly to the presence of obstruction. This obstruction may be measured (in millimeters of mercury [mm Hg]), either noninvasively with Doppler echocardiography, or by cardiac catheterization, which determines pressure measurements directly, using catheters that are introduced into the heart via arm vessels.

Obstruction essentially means the *difference* in pressure *(or the pressure gradient)* between the left ventricle and aorta. It is also important for patients to realize that obstruction in HCM may change spontaneously in degree – from day-to-day or even hour-to-hour, with exercise or emotion, or after meals or alcohol consumption. Therefore, patients should consider the actual numerical value for the gradient at any given time in light of its dynamic nature and potential changes, and not necessarily as a fixed (or "hard") number.

Heart Function in HCM

The thickened muscle in HCM usually contracts well in the presence of small or normal-sized heart chambers – sometimes, better than normal – and ejects most of the blood very rapidly from the heart (i.e., in systole); only a very few patients develop depressed contraction and severe heart failure (as will be discussed later). However, the heart muscle in HCM is often stiff and relaxes poorly when blood enters the ventricles passively during diastole. It is believed that most symptoms in HCM (such as shortness of breath with exercise) are related, at least in part, to this impaired filling of the ventricles. This type of "heart failure" characteristic of HCM is very different from the more usual situation in the failing heart, which involves dilatation of the ventricles and poor contractile function.

Ischemia, or impaired blood flow to the heart muscle, may also be responsible for symptoms (including chest pain) in HCM. This ischemia may be similar in some respects to that experienced by patients with coronary artery disease due to atherosclerosis (with plaque in the large coronary arteries); in HCM, it is expressed either as true angina pectoris (relatively short-lasting pain or pressure in the center of the chest associated with exertion, or occurring after meals), or "atypical" pain patterns that differ from classic angina in a variety of ways. In HCM, ischemia occurs by completely different mechanisms than in coronary artery disease, and is probably caused by small arteries *within* the heart muscle which are abnormal by virtue of thickened walls and small openings. It is also possible that ischemia results in part because the heart muscle is too thick for the available blood supply. Unfortunately, the identification of ischemia in HCM with testing is difficult and often unreliable, and, therefore, precise assessment of this problem in patients has been a challenge. Moreover, ischemia can have adverse consequences because it may cause heart cells to die and be replaced by scars.

When Does HCM Develop? HCM in Infants and Children

Since HCM is a genetic disease, the mutant gene is present from conception and all affected family members carry exactly the same mutation. While the hypertrophy, as visualized with the echocardiogram, occasionally may be present at birth or in very young children, it is much more common for the heart to appear normal until about age 12 in genetically affected family members.

Usually (as described in detail later), hypertrophy develops in association with accelerated growth and is apparent on the echocardiogram in the teenage years (by about age 15). For the vast majority of patients, there does not appear to be significant change in muscle thickness after age 18.

In fact, HCM is identified rather uncommonly in children, and therefore represents, to the pediatric cardiologist, a rare disease. HCM, in most affected children, is initially suspected by a heart murmur, transient symptoms, abnormal electrocardiogram, family history of HCM, or sometimes by preparticipation screening for competitive athletics; the diagnosis is later confirmed by echocardiography. The percentage of children with HCM who have important and limiting symptoms is small, and the occurrence of sudden unexpected death before age 10 is believed to be exceedingly uncommon.

Indeed, the diagnosis of HCM in children and adolescents (particularly if asymptomatic) often represents a major dilemma for pediatric cardiologists since the patients are so young and predictions regarding future prognosis are therefore much more difficult. It is possible for such circumstances to lead to overreaction and there is occasionally a tendency to pursue major interventions, perhaps prematurely. Very rarely, HCM presents during infancy with heart failure; this appears to be a particularly unfavorable development and many of these children die early in life despite aggressive drug therapy. On the other hand, most infants or young children (less than 4 years old) with thick hearts usually do not have traditional HCM but, often, a number of other conditions in which the heart manifestations can mimic HCM: most commonly, Noonan's syndrome, glycogen storage disease, Friedreich's ataxia, or symptoms related to the presence of diabetes in the mother during pregnancy (a situation in which the hypertrophy quickly disappears spontaneously).

What Are the Symptoms of HCM?

It is important to realize that HCM is an unusual disease, in that it can affect people at virtually any age. HCM-related symptoms may develop in patients from infancy (as young as 1 day old) to later life (as old as 90 years of age, or older), although this is uncommon during the first 10 years. The symptoms of HCM are generally similar to other forms of heart disease and there is no particular complaint that is unique to HCM. With respect to the symptoms of shortness of breath or chest pain, patients often relate "good and bad days" during which such symptoms may be perceived as quite different in degree. The precise basis for this variability is uncertain. However, when relating symptoms to their doctors, it is important that patients not limit their histories to either the best or worst, but rather provide the full spectrum of complaints that they have experienced.

Shortness of Breath

Exercise capacity may be limited by shortness of breath and fatigue (also called *dyspnea*). Most individuals experience only mild limitation of exercise, but occasionally this becomes severe and patients are unable to walk even one city block or a flight of stairs without stopping due to shortness of breath; a small minority may have shortness of breath at rest.

Chest Pain

Chest pain or pressure (sometimes called *angina*) is a common symptom. It is usually brought on by exertion or meals and relieved by rest, but may also occur at rest. In HCM, chest discomfort may also take different forms – sharp or dull, in the center of the chest or elsewhere, or prolonged and unrelated to exertion. The cause of the pain is thought to be insufficient oxygen supply to the heart muscle. In HCM, the main coronary arteries are usually free of significant plaque or narrowing from atherosclerosis. In contrast, the smaller arteries within the heart muscle are often narrowed; the greatly thickened left ventricular muscle demands an increased oxygen supply that often cannot be served by the abnormal small arteries.

Fatigue

Fatigue is a complaint that is distinctive from shortness of breath with exertion; many patients complain of excessive tiredness, either related or unrelated to exertion.

Palpitations

Patients may occasionally feel an extra or skipped beat, and this may be normal. Sometimes, however, such an awareness of the beating heart is indicative of an irregular heart rhythm. This symptom, ***palpitations***, may also occur commonly in other forms of heart disease, and even in many normal people. Palpitations begin suddenly, and may be associated with symptoms such as sweating or lightheadedness. Such episodes should be reported to the cardiologist for further investigation.

Lightheadedness and Fainting

Patients with HCM may experience impairment or loss of consciousness, i.e., lightheadedness or dizziness, and, more seriously, fainting (known as ***syncope***). Such episodes may occur in association with exercise, or without apparent provocation, and the reason for these events is not always clear, even after testing. Impaired consciousness may be due to an irregularity of the heartbeat, a fall in blood pressure; very uncommonly, it is unrelated to HCM and heart disease, and is termed "simple faint" or vasovagal syncope, in which the vagus nerve is excessively active. Fainting (or near-fainting) should be reported immediately to the cardiologist and investigated. Unfortunately, such episodes represent the most difficult HCM symptom to evaluate, simply because the events occur without warning, and are usually long over before the physician can order tests to investigate their origin.

HCM and the Physical Examination

In many patients with HCM, the physical examination is unremarkable, and either no or only a soft heart murmur is present. This fact is surprising to many people, but only reflects the fact that under resting conditions, most HCM patients do not have outflow obstruction (and the murmur in this disease is produced by obstruction). The infrequency of loud heart murmurs in HCM is responsible, in part, for the difficulty in identifying the disease during routine preparticipation sports screening.

Most HCM patients (particularly young people) have a strong heart impulse that can be felt on the left side of the chest, which reflects the thickened and forcibly contracting heart. The observation of a forcibly beating heart may trigger recognition of HCM in some instances, even in the absence of a heart murmur. When present, the most obvious finding on physical examination is a systolic heart murmur. Such murmurs usually indicate partial obstruction to blood flow out of the left side of the heart, and may change spontaneously throughout the day, and with activity. The cardiologist may also be able to provoke a heart murmur by asking the patient to change body position (i.e., to stand) or undergo maneuvers such as holding one's breath and straining (Valsalva maneuver), inhaling amyl nitrite, or exercising. Such a finding indicates the development of outflow obstruction *under provocable conditions* and is very common in HCM. In general, however, the presence of a murmur is not often a particularly unfavorable sign; it simply indicates the presence of obstruction or mitral regurgitation.

How Is HCM Diagnosed and Which Tests Are Used?

Echocardiogram

The primary test for the clinical diagnosis of HCM is an ultrasound scan of the heart called an ***echocardiogram***. This is an entirely safe noninvasive test which produces a two-dimensional image of the heart that is viewed in real-time, and is recorded on a standard VHS videotape, along with single-dimension views (called the M-mode echocardiogram) (Figures 7 and 8). The echocardiogram is performed by a specially trained technologist (the cardiologist may also be present during the test) who places a transducer and a small amount of transmitting gel on the chest to generate images of the heart in several cross-sections (Figure 8). From the echocardiographic images, the excessive thickness of the muscle (i.e., left ventricular wall) can be easily measured. An additional ultrasound mode called ***Doppler*** is very useful and includes a color-coded image of blood flow within the heart. Turbulent flow and the degree of obstruction (if present), as well as valve leakage (mitral regurgitation), can be detected and measured with precision. Therefore, the echocardiogram can provide a thorough structural and functional assessment of HCM, largely avoiding invasive procedures such as cardiac catheterization.

Electrocardiogram

The standard electrocardiogram (ECG, also known as the 12-lead ECG) is performed by placing electrodes on the chest, wrists, and ankles

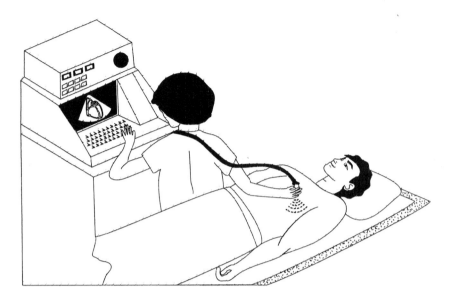

Figure 8. The clinical diagnosis of HCM is generally made with an ultrasound scan of the heart called an echocardiogram (or echo, for short). Like the ECG, this is an entirely safe and pain-free test that produces a picture of the heart, so that the excessive thickness of the heart muscle wall characteristic of HCM can be easily measured.

and records the electrical signals from the heart. In HCM, the ECG usually shows a variety of abnormal electrical signals due to the muscle thickening. In a minority of HCM patients (about 5%), the ECG may be normal or show particularly minor alterations. ECG abnormalities are also not specific to HCM and may be found in many other heart conditions. In fact, the abnormal ECG in HCM can mimic that of a previous (healed) myocardial infarction; some HCM patients have been advised erroneously that they have previously experienced a "heart attack" (which is a term that literally refers only to the consequence of coronary artery disease).

Other Diagnostic Tests

While two-dimensional echocardiography is the principal clinical test for the diagnosis of HCM, other tests have been used selectively for this purpose. For example, nuclear magnetic resonance (NMR), based on magnet technology, may provide extremely high-quality images of the heart, which are often superior to echocardiography. However, NMR scanners (adjusted to use for the heart) are uncommon and generally confined to research centers, and they are extremely expensive, rendering the tests quite costly to patients. Also, obese patients and those with implanted devices or claustrophobia may not be suitable candidates for NMR. However, an NMR test could be a useful diagnostic aid in selected patients, including those with unsatisfactory or ambiguous echocardiographic studies.

Laboratory DNA analysis (of blood or other tissue) is, of course, the most definitive method for making the diagnosis of HCM. However, such genetic analysis is not, at present, routinely available on a clinical basis. Most successful genotyping has been achieved through selected participation in a research project.

Other Investigations that May Be Useful

Additional investigations may be required in selected patients to assess HCM.

Cardiac Catheterization

With the widespread use of echocardiography and Doppler imaging, the cardiac catheterization procedure is rarely performed to evaluate HCM, except perhaps prior to surgery or to exclude associated coronary artery disease. With *cardiac catheterization,* a fine tube is passed through a vein (usually in the groin) to the heart using x-ray guidance. Pressures within the heart chambers are then measured, and an *angiogram* (x-ray) of the heart is obtained by the injection of dye to assess mitral regurgitation, contraction of the left ventricle, or narrowing of the coronary arteries by plaque. With the advent of echocardiography, there is no longer any reason to perform multiple cardiac catheterization procedures in this disease. However, because it is possible for HCM patients over the age of 40 with chest pain to have both coronary artery disease and HCM, it may be necessary in some circumstances to perform a cardiac catheterization, to define the anatomy of the coronary arteries (by injecting contrast dye directly).

Electrophysiological Studies

This is a specialized form of cardiac catheterization which has been performed selectively to define the risk of electrical instability which may predispose to sudden death. *Electrophysiological studies* involve the passage of fine wires from the veins in the groin, arm, or shoulder into the heart under x-ray guidance. These wires are then used to make measurements or apply stimuli to record the response of the electrical system of the heart. Sometimes, irregularities of the heartbeat (otherwise known as ***arrhythmias***) are intentionally provoked in the laboratory (and immediately terminated) to estimate the predisposition to develop such rhythms naturally. At present, most investigators believe that electrophysiological testing is informative for assessing risk for sudden death only in selected patients.

Exercise Testing

The severity of exercise limitation and the effect of treatment can be assessed with bicycle or treadmill ***exercise testing***. Exercise testing can also provide an objective measurement of improvement, stability, or deterioration over time. The exercise test can be combined with an echocardiogram (stress echocardiogram) to evaluate heart wall motion with exertion. Also, if blood pressure drops or fails to increase appropriately during exercise, this may indicate an important instability and is considered a risk factor.

Ambulatory Holter Monitoring

This test is a noninvasive and continuous *ambulatory* recording of the heartbeat over 24 or 48 hours during normal activities. A Holter monitor is a simple and safe test that will detect potentially important irregularities of the heartbeat of which the patient may be unaware.

Radionuclide Studies

In these tests, substances producing very tiny (safe) amounts of radioactivity are injected into the bloodstream to create a heart scan. These tests are occasionally performed in HCM patients to assess the contraction and filling of the ventricles, at rest and with exercise.

General Outlook for Patients with HCM

The severity of symptoms and risk of complications varies greatly between HCM patients, and it should be emphasized that many people never experience serious problems related to their disease. Indeed, HCM is compatible with normal longevity and elderly patients, in their 70s and 80s, are not uncommon, including some in their 90s. When considering the *overall* population of adult patients with HCM, this disease may not significantly increase an individual patient's risk (over the known risks of living, such as cancer, coronary heart disease, or accidents) and may not limit considerably the quality or duration of life (Figure 9). The most accurate mortality rate for the overall disease is about 1% per year, which means that each year 1 of 100 patients may die for a reason directly related to their disease.

On the other hand, some patients do experience significant symptoms and/or disability, or may be at risk for premature death. There are three circumstances in which patients with HCM die prematurely: (1) suddenly and unexpectedly, often in the younger patients; (2) related to severe progressive heart failure, usually in mid-life; and (3) due to stroke, usually in older patients with atrial fibrillation. Disabling symptoms (usually shortness of breath and/or chest pain with exertion), whether mild or more severe, may remain stable throughout much of adult life, or deteriorate and require a major intervention. Each patient with HCM, however, must be assessed individually to determine the subgroup of patients to which they most likely belong, e.g., high or low risk for sudden death, or predisposition to progressive symptoms, or atrial fibrillation.

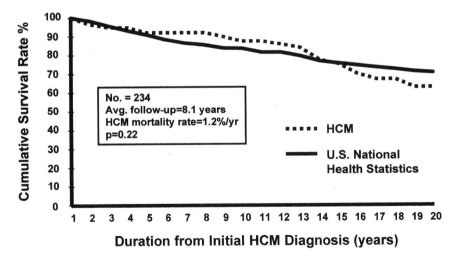

Figure 9. Mortality in a regional HCM population from the upper Midwest compared to that in the general U.S. population due to all causes (e.g., cancer, homicide, coronary heart disease, etc.). The two populations are not different in terms of total mortality. *Therefore, HCM itself does not add to the overall risk of living.*

Therefore, it is an important general principle regarding HCM that all patients are *not* the same in terms of prognosis, clinical presentation, or determination of appropriate treatment (Figure 10). There are several different clinical profiles that patients may present, and it is important not to "lump" all these together under the homogeneous label of HCM. Many patients have virtually no risk associated with their disease and some deserve high-risk status. *However, the overall disease is not, per se, a high-risk condition, and HCM should not be regarded as a uniformly unfavorable disease.* Obviously, this volume can provide only a broad overview of the prognosis for HCM patients and is not a substitute for the careful evaluation of an individual patient by a cardiologist who is knowledgeable about this disease.

Complications of HCM

Arrhythmias

A variety of arrhythmias, or irregularities of the heartbeat, are exceedingly common in patients with HCM and are often detected by exercise testing or Holter monitoring. Prolonged arrhythmias known

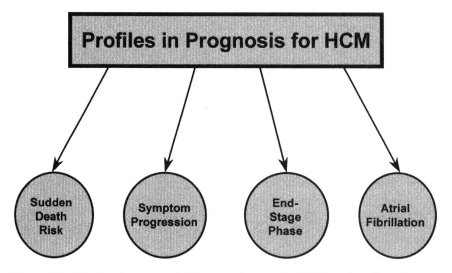

Figure 10. *Profiles in prognosis.* Many patients with HCM can be placed in one of these categories for the purposes of judging the prognosis, as well as for eventually formulating treatment strategies. This diagram emphasizes the necessity of viewing HCM in terms of such subgroups so that treatment can be tailored to particular clinical profiles, with the proper selection of patients.

as *ventricular tachycardia* or *atrial fibrillation* are particularly important and require treatment in the vast majority of cases. Transient arrhythmias with premature beats from the atria and ventricles occur much more commonly, but usually do not have the same importance to patients, even when present in large numbers.

Ventricular Tachycardia

Ventricular tachycardia is an incessant and repetitive occurrence of abnormal beats arising from the ventricles. This is a potentially serious arrhythmia in HCM since it may lead to ventricular fibrillation and sudden death. Patients prone to this arrhythmia may be treated with an implantable cardioverter-defibrillator, as will be discussed later.

Congestive Heart Failure

Any HCM patient with significant shortness of breath during physical exertion is, strictly speaking, experiencing a degree of heart failure. However, this is a different form of heart failure than that which occurs in coronary artery disease, or many other cardiac conditions; in HCM, congestive failure is paradoxically present in a heart which is not dilated (enlarged) and shows normal contraction of the ventricles. In other diseases heart failure is a profound condition, usually occurring after a myocardial infarction ("heart attack"), and producing dilated ventricles that contract poorly. Occasionally, heart failure in HCM may become intractable and fail to respond further to drugs, requiring major therapy and intervention.

Atrial Fibrillation and Stroke

With atrial fibrillation, the normal regular heart rhythm is altered due to loss of the normal contraction of the atria (the two upper chambers), causing the ventricles to beat in an irregular rhythm. Atrial fibrillation may be episodic (i.e., paroxysmal) or persistent (i.e., chronic) and occurs in as much as 20-25% of HCM patients, and is often responsible for important symptoms of heart failure at that time. While some patients are unaware of their atrial fibrillation, most rapidly develop symptoms such as shortness of breath, dizziness, and fainting. Atrial fibrillation increases in frequency with age, but may occur at any time in adulthood (after about 30-35 years of age). Although all the potential long-term consequences of atrial fibrillation are not completely resolved, this arrhythmia does not seem to be associated with increased risk for sudden death.

Because the atria "fibrillate" there is also a direct link and risk for clot formation due to the stagnant blood flow. This can result in a stroke if the blood clot travels to the brain. The risk of such an event in HCM is about 1% per year. Anticoagulation, to protect against stroke, is important, and the pros and cons of this treatment should be discussed in detail by the patient and cardiologist.

Sometimes atrial fibrillation will revert to normal rhythm spontaneously, but patients often require drug treatment to abolish the abnormal rhythm or to control and reduce the rapid ventricular rate (if the patient must remain in atrial fibrillation). However, *electrical cardioversion* may be used to convert the heart back to its normal rhythm. This treatment requires admission to the hospital and consists of applying a small electrical shock to the chest. Atrial fibrillation occurs in forms of heart disease other than HCM (or even in patients without heart disease), is relatively common in HCM, occurring in up to 20% of patients, and increases in occurrence with age.

The Problem of Sudden Death

Since the first description of HCM over 40 years ago, the issue of risk for sudden and unexpected death has been a highly visible issue. In reality, only a small proportion of patients with HCM are at increased risk for sudden premature death due to arrhythmias, which usually occur with little or no warning (Figure 11). The magnitude of this particular problem among all HCM patients has probably been exaggerated over the years due to the disproportionate number of reports from institutions in which there was the preferential referral of high-risk patients (i.e., so-called tertiary centers).

Nevertheless, sudden unexpected collapse remains a devastating consideration for many patients living with this disease. We know that sudden death clearly occurs most commonly in young people (30 years of age or younger), but on the other hand there is no particular age group which is immune, and sudden deaths have been reported in midlife and beyond. The first 10 to 12 years of life are generally free of adverse events such as sudden death (at a time when hypertrophy is also usually absent), but a very few virulent cases in young children have been reported, with substantial hypertrophy or sudden death.

Sudden death may occur in some susceptible patients with HCM because the abnormal heart muscle in HCM can sometimes interfere

HCM: identification of high risk patients

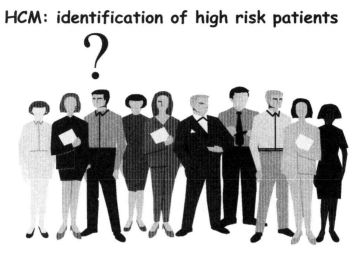

Figure 11. While the risk for sudden death in young people has been made a highly visible feature of HCM, in reality it is an uncommon occurrence and only a minority of HCM patients is truly at risk. Therefore, an important objective of the HCM evaluation is to identify which patients, among all those with this condition, appear to be at particularly high risk.

with normal electrical activity. For example, in those portions of the left ventricular wall with abnormal architecture and myocyte disarray, the electrical signal may become unstable as it crosses areas of scarring and disorganized cells. This can, in turn, lead to distorted electrical impulses that generate fast or erratic heart rhythms, some of which can lead to adverse clinical events (Figures 1 and 12).

At present, the highest risk for sudden death appears to be most associated with one or more of the following features of the disease (i.e., risk factors) (Figure 13): prior cardiac arrest (heart stoppage or prolonged ventricular arrhythmia); fainting, particularly when repetitive or associated with exertion or when it occurs in young people; serious arrhythmias (such as ventricular tachycardia) repeatedly detected by Holter monitoring; family history of HCM-related premature sudden death in one or more close relatives; or extreme increase in the thickness of the left ventricular wall. The latter disease feature applies to an important 10% of all HCM patients in whom the maximum thickness of the left ventricular wall is 3.0 centimeters (i.e., 30 millimeters) or more, and who may therefore be at increased risk based soley on their particular heart structure (Figures 7 and 14).

On the other hand, and deserving of equal emphasis, most patients with HCM are without risk factors for sudden death and are at low risk for premature death, and therefore should receive a large measure of reassurance in this regard.

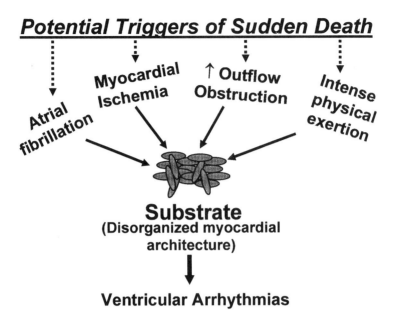

Figure 12. Proposed mechanism by which myocardial disarray (as the "substrate") may result in serious ventricular arrhythmias, when activated by a variety of potential "triggers" that may either be parts of the HCM disease process, or environmental factors such as intense physical exertion in certain susceptible individuals. ↑ = increased.

Endocarditis

Endocarditis is an infection of the heart which occurs very uncommonly in HCM. Nevertheless, it is important to be protected from the unlikely occurrence of endocarditis since this complication can cause severe tissue damage of the heart valve, sometimes necessitating valve replacement. Bacteria which gain access to the bloodstream can stick to the inside of the heart (specifically, on the mitral valve in HCM) after it has been roughened by turbulent blood flow. The risk of bacterial endocarditis in HCM seems to be limited to those patients with the obstructive form.

Athletes and HCM

While sudden death is very uncommon among HCM patients as a group, HCM is, on the other hand, the most frequent cause of death among young persons (younger than age 35) who die suddenly and

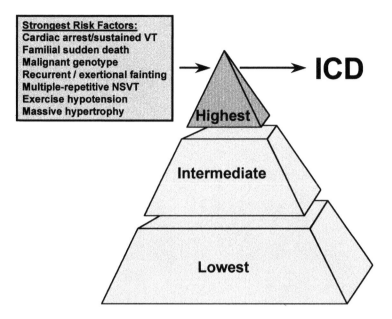

Strongest Risk Factors:
Cardiac arrest/sustained VT
Familial sudden death
Malignant genotype
Recurrent / exertional fainting
Multiple-repetitive NSVT
Exercise hypotension
Massive hypertrophy

Figure 13. *The HCM disease features that give a patient high-risk status.* The presence of one or more of these clinical risk factors is sufficient to justify consideration of treatment to prevent sudden death, probably with an implantable defibrillator (ICD). VT = ventricular tachycardia; NSVT = nonsustained (lasting only a few beats) ventricular tachycardia on Holter monitoring.

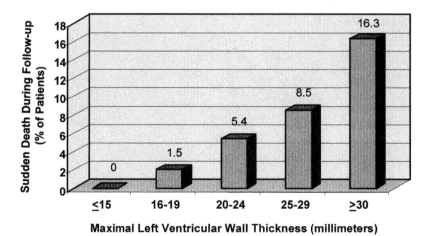

Figure 14. *Relation between the degree to which the left ventricular wall is thickened and the likelihood of sudden death.* This analysis shows little risk associated with mild degrees of thickening, but extreme increases in wall thickness (30 millimeters or more) convey a much greater risk.

unexpectedly (Figures 15 and 16). This also includes young participants in competitive sports who die suddenly on the athletic field, for whom HCM is the single most common cause (in about one-third) – although many other congenital disorders may also be responsible for these tragedies. In fact, an important percentage of HCM-related sudden death in youths occurs during physical exertion whether the individuals are athletes or not. Based on these facts, it seems most prudent (and has become a standard recommendation) that young people withdraw from intense competitive athletics once the diagnosis of HCM has been determined. This applies to most sports, particularly those involving burst exertion and sprinting, but participation in a few low-intensity sports, such as golf and bowling, is not felt to pose significant risk. It is believed that competitive athletics and a lifestyle involving intense physical activity add to the risks of HCM, and that removal from such athletic activities (which by their competitive nature do not easily permit the athlete to withdraw should cardiac symptoms be perceived) will restore that individual to more acceptable risk levels. Recommendations concerning the criteria that should be used for sports eligibility and disqualification with cardiovascular disease have been formalized in a document known as Bethesda Conference #26, sponsored by the

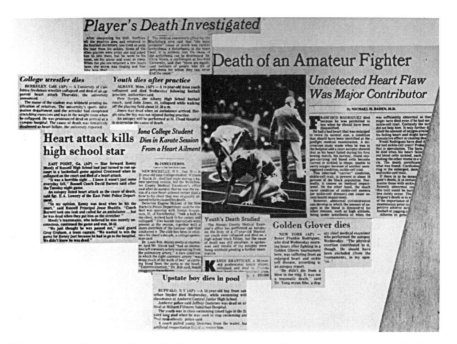

Figure 15. Athletic field deaths in young sports participants have achieved a high level of public visibility. HCM is the single most common cause of these deaths.

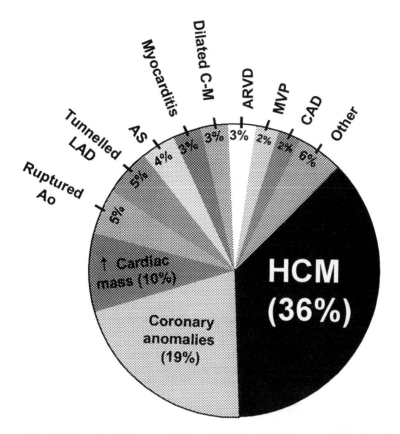

Figure 16. *Sudden death in young trained athletes.* HCM accounts for about one-third of these tragic events. Several other (mostly congenital) forms of heart disease shown here can also be responsible for these deaths in young people. Ao = aorta; LAD = left anterior descending coronary artery; AS = aortic stenosis; C-M = cardiomyopathy; ARVD = arrhythmogenic right ventricular dysplasia; MVP = mitral valve prolapse; CAD = coronary artery disease (due to atherosclerosis). ↑ = increased.

American College of Cardiology (Bethesda, MD) and published in the *Journal of the American College of Cardiology* in 1994.

Some normal, trained athletes with hypertrophy (i.e., wall thickening) of the left ventricle, resulting from intense and prolonged athletic training, may resemble HCM structurally (i.e., as evident on an echocardiogram). The distinction between the two may be difficult to make in some such athletes, but often can be resolved with noninvasive testing. It is obviously an important distinction since HCM can have important ramifications, while changes in heart structure produced by athletic training alone are not believed to represent a true (pathologic) abnormality or to have important clinical consequences to patients.

Special Considerations: Gender and Race

HCM has been reported in published articles to be more common in men than in women (about 60:40). In reality, because HCM is a genetic disease transmitted as an autosomal dominant trait, it occurs equally in men and women. This indicates that HCM is *diagnosed* less frequently in women than men. The reasons for this phenomenon are uncertain. However, there is now some evidence that women with HCM develop symptoms and are diagnosed later, and may have more severe consequences from their disease, than men.

HCM has rarely been diagnosed in African-Americans in the clinical setting. On the other hand, HCM has proved to be a common cause of sudden death in young, male African-American athletes (who did not have an HCM diagnosis or cardiovascular evaluation prior to death). This suggests that the rarity of the HCM diagnosis in young African-Americans may be related, in large part, to socioeconomic factors that create limited access to medical specialists, which is a prerequisite for obtaining an echocardiogram and the clinical diagnosis of HCM.

Treatment

There are several forms of treatment available that are directed toward improving heart function, relieving symptoms. and preventing complications in HCM patients. Many individuals who have very mild or no symptoms do not require treatment, unless they are judged to be at high-risk for sudden death. For those patients who do require therapy, one or more of the following treatment strategies should be considered.

Drugs

Drugs (medications) are usually the first line of treatment for patients with shortness of breath or chest pain associated with exertion. Many patients realize benefit from medications, with reduction in their symptoms. A variety of drugs are currently used in treating HCM and new drugs are likely to become available in the future. The need for drug treatment and the precise choice of medication has to be made on an individual basis and may need to be modified for any patient over time. Children may develop such symptoms, though uncommonly, and they are treated with the same drugs, and largely in the same fashion, as adults. The most commonly used drugs are described below.

Beta-Blockers

Beta-blockers slow the heartbeat and probably improve filling of the ventricles in diastole, reduce the force of contraction, and may also decrease obstruction during exercise. These drugs are also widely used in medical practice for other types of heart disease, including high blood pressure. Sometimes, these drugs can produce excessive fatigue, nightmares, and impotence. Several beta-blockers have been used in HCM. The most common are: propranolol (Inderal®), and drugs such as atenolol (Tenormin®), nadolol (Corgard®) and metoprolol (Lopressor®). Long-acting preparations of these drugs are now used extensively and usually require a single dose daily.

Calcium Channel Blockers

The second major group of drugs used are the calcium channel blockers; verapamil (Calan®; Isoptin®) is most commonly administered in HCM. This drug appears to relax the heart and improve filling of the ventricles (during diastole). Also, like beta-blockers, verapamil can cause excessive slowing of the heart rate and lower blood pressure, and some patients complain of constipation. Beta-blockers and verapamil should not be administered together. Another calcium blocker, diltiazem (Cardizem®), has also been used occasionally in HCM.

Disopyramide

Disopyramide (Norpace®) relaxes the heart and is also an antiarrhythmic agent. It has been used somewhat less commonly than beta-blockers and verapamil as a drug to treat HCM patients with symptoms.

Antiarrhythmic Drugs

These drugs might be used when an arrhythmia such as ventricular tachycardia or atrial fibrillation is detected and judged to be an important risk to an individual patient. Amiodarone (Cordarone®; Pacerone®) is the most commonly used antiarrhythmic drug in HCM, either to reduce the chances of recurrent atrial fibrillation or, at some centers, to reduce the risk of sudden death. However, amiodarone does have several potential side effects, especially sensitivity to sunlight (which can be avoided with use of barrier creams that act as sunblocks), reversible effects on the thyroid gland, and occasionally, damage to the lungs or liver. For these reasons, it is always uncertain whether amiodarone can be tolerated for particularly long periods of time in any individual patient, particularly those young people at high risk for sudden death. Some cardiologists have used the antiarrhythmic drug, *sotolol,* which also contains a beta-blocker. Other antiarrhythmic drugs such as quinidine and procainamide have been abandoned due to their ability to induce important arrhythmias.

Diuretics

Some severely symptomatic patients develop fluid retention, and in this situation, ***diuretics*** (water tablets), which increase urine flow, may be administered.

Anticoagulants

Most patients with episodic or persistent atrial fibrillation should take anticoagulants ("blood thinners"; usually warfarin) to prevent stroke, which may result if a clot forms in the atria and a portion breaks off and travels through the arterial blood stream to the brain. Such treatment requires monitoring with a blood test, approximately on a monthly basis. Given the potential complications of anticoagulation (i.e., brain hemorrhage as a consequence of trauma), the decision of whether to begin anticoagulants may be a difficult one and obviously should be made in close consultation with the cardiologist.

Antibiotics

Although ***endocarditis*** is rare, patients with the obstructive form of HCM and turbulent blood flow in the left ventricular outflow tract should receive ***antibiotic prophylaxis*** prior to any dental procedures (including cleaning) or other surgical interventions. The American Heart Association recommendation for bacterial endocarditis prophylaxis is: amoxicillin (2 grams for adults; 50 milligrams per kilogram for children) orally 1 hour before the procedure. Arrangements for antibiotic prophylaxis should be made directly with the dentist or surgeon when making the appointment, well in advance of the procedure.

Implantable Defibrillators

Those HCM patients clearly at high-risk for sudden death may be candidates for an ***implantable cardioverter-defibrillator (ICD)***, a sophisticated device which is permanently implanted internally. The ICD has the capability of sensing potentially lethal arrhythmias and then introducing a shock (or antitachycardia pacing) to terminate these arrhythmias and to restore normal heart rhythm (Figures 17 and 18).

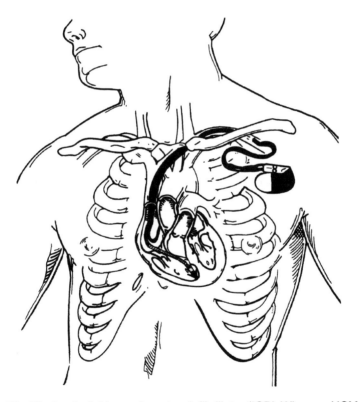

Figure 17. *The implantable cardioverter-defibrillator (ICD).* When an HCM patient is judged to be at high risk, this device can be permanently implanted to automatically detect and terminate arrhythmias that can be lethal. A small box about the size of a pacemaker is placed under the skin just below the clavicle, and is attached to wires (called leads) introduced into the heart. These wires are responsible for sensing (and recording) the heart rhythm and delivering the shock, if necessary, that restores normal electrical activity.

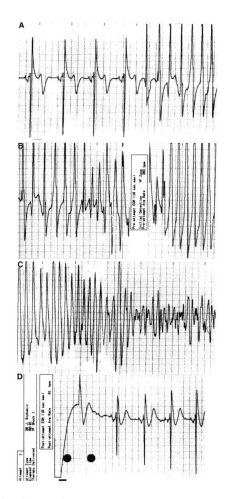

Figure 18. *ICD aborting sudden death.* This is a continuous recording of an electrocardiogram obtained by the recording system of the ICD at the time of a life-saving event in a 36-year-old man with HCM. This patient, who had not previously experienced symptoms, received his ICD prophylactically because of high-risk status: he had extreme left ventricular wall thickening and his younger brother had recently died suddenly of HCM. For almost 5 years, nothing at all occurred. Then, early one morning while he was asleep at 1:00 A.M., normal heart rhythm converted suddenly to a life-threatening rhythm disturbance known as ventricular tachycardia (panel **A**). In panel **B**, ventricular tachycardia continues, and this is sensed by the device (note the box indicating the ICD is charging). While the device is charging, in panel **C**, the situation deteriorates with ventricular tachycardia converting to a particularly serious rhythm known as ventricular fibrillation in which the ventricles (two lower chambers) fibrillate and do not contract effectively to sustain a measurable blood pressure. In panel **D**, the ICD automatically delivers a shock (denoted by the box at lower left), which immediately converts the patient to a normal heart rhythm. Other than being awakened abruptly by the shock, the patient experienced no difficulties then, or in the ensuing 4 years.

At the same time, an ECG recording is generated directly by the device to precisely document the event. Recently, there has been much more experience with, and interest in, the ICD for high-risk patients with HCM, and we believe this device has favorably changed the clinical course of the disease for many patients. In one study (Figure 19), the ICD automatically and appropriately intervened, aborting potentially lethal arrhythmias in individual high-risk patients at a rate of 7% per year (which could amount to more than 50% in 10 years, based on conservative extrapolation). The rate of discharge (of shocks) was highest if the ICD was implanted because of a prior cardiac arrest (11% per year); the shock rate was also substantial, however, in those patients for whom the device was used because of one or more of the aforementioned risk factors but without a prior major clinical event (about 5% per year). Of note, most of these latter patients were young and without symptoms.

Also, over the last few years these devices have become smaller and much easier to implant in unobtrusive positions on the chest, requiring in most instances only an overnight hospital stay without major surgery. The ICD leads can be introduced through the veins (and are therefore present inside the heart chamber) and the generator is

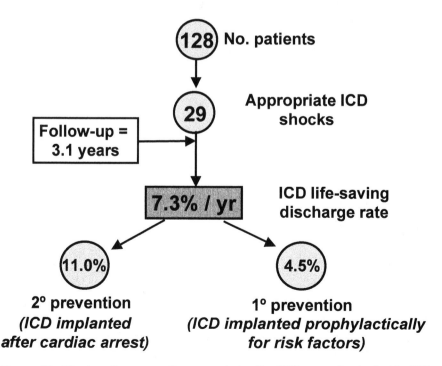

Figure 19. The results, over a 3-year period, after ICDs were implanted in 128 high-risk patients with HCM.

placed just under the clavicle. Even a few high-risk children (younger than 16 years old) have now had ICDs implanted.

Patients must also be aware of the possible complications associated with ICDs, such as false shocks due to fast heart rates that are actually benign (in up to 25% of patients, at present). Furthermore, there is a small chance of infection, and problems with the leads (usually related to breakage) are not uncommon.

As the risk period in HCM is characteristically very long (theoretically 20-50 years in some patients), the ICD is likely to be a long-term or lifelong treatment, thereby creating the crucial necessity for careful and consistent maintenance and interrogation of the device (usually 4 times per year) including regular battery replacement (at approximately 5 to 7 year intervals, but possibly up to about 8 years, depending on usage). We have knowledge of several HCM patients in whom the ICD discharged appropriately for the first time as long as 4 to 9 years after it was implanted, emphasizing the unpredictable timing of these events.

In the future, we expect that ICDs will be offered as life-saving protection to many more HCM patients, either after they have already survived a life-threatening event such as cardiac arrest or, prophylactically, because they have a high-risk status (with the aforementioned risk factors such as a family history of HCM-related sudden death in a close relative), i.e., *before* any major problems occur, such as cardiac arrest. However, it is important to note the ICD is *not* a treatment intended for all HCM patients, but only for those who are judged by their cardiologist to be truly at high risk. Indeed, it should be emphasized that most HCM patients are at low (or no) risk for sudden death, including (but not limited to) those with only mild thickening of the heart wall and those without a family history of sudden death. In high-risk patients there does not seem at present to be much use for antiarrhythmic drugs (such as amiodarone) as alternatives to the ICD, since these medications have not been proven to be completely effective in these circumstances, and may also have important side effects over the long term.

Surgery

Surgery (***ventricular septal myotomy-myectomy***) is reserved for those patients with marked outflow obstruction who have severe symptoms that are unresponsive to drugs or other treatment (Figure 20). Specifically, surgery is the preferred treatment in those patients with obstructive gradients (of 50 millimeters of mercury [mm Hg] or more] and symptoms that persist even after all drugs or other options have

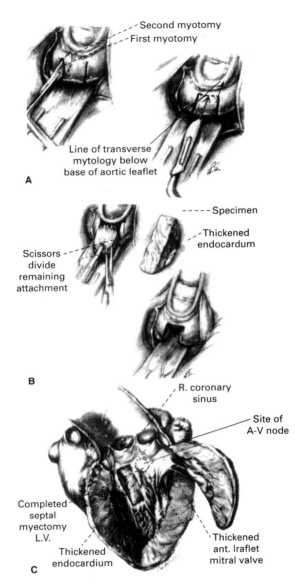

Figure 20. Surgery in HCM (the ventricular septal myotomy-myectomy operation; Morrow procedure). After the patient is placed under cardiopulmonary bypass, the surgeon opens the aorta and performs surgery through that exposure. **(A)** First, two vertical parallel incisions are made in the top portion of the ventricular septum. A third incision is then made, connecting the two parallel incisions. **(B)** This section of muscle is then removed. **(C)** At completion of the myotomy-myectomy, a rectangular channel is evident extending from just below the aortic valve to a point just beyond where obstruction occurs (where the mitral valve contacts the septum). It should be emphasized that the surgeon does not, in fact, open the left ventricle as shown here for illustrative purposes only.

been exhausted. Several surgical techniques have been used in HCM, but the one which is most accepted is the ventricular septal myotomy-myectomy operation in which the surgeon removes a small portion of the thickened muscle from the upper portion of ventricular septum, thereby widening the left ventricular cavity in that region and relieving the obstruction.

Surgery for HCM should be performed only by surgeons who are sufficiently experienced with this operation (usually at tertiary referral institutions); therefore, having performed myotomy-myectomy only a few times is probably not sufficient. This has created a situation where HCM patients requiring surgery have frequently traveled outside of their home communities for treatment. In experienced centers, operative mortality is now rather low (2% or less and less than 1% in some), with most patients reporting a long-lasting and measurable improvement in symptoms after operation. Surgery can be (and has been) performed safely in children and older patients with HCM. Operative risk for HCM appears to be increased only if additional heart surgery (such as coronary artery bypass grafting) must also be performed at the same time.

If the operation is performed properly, obstruction under resting conditions will be virtually abolished and will not return. Occasionally, in selected patients, instead of a ventricular septal myotomy-myectomy, the surgeon may choose to replace the mitral valve with an artificial valve. There is no reason to perform both a myectomy and a valve replacement.

Of course, some patients who meet the clinical criteria for surgery are not, in fact, optimal candidates for operation, either because of other complicating diseases, geographical inaccessibility to an experienced surgeon, disability from other complicating diseases, advanced age, lack of motivation on the part of the patient, or other factors. Indeed, these issues are fundamental to any consideration of alternatives to myotomy-myectomy surgery.

Alcohol Septal Ablation (Nonsurgical Myectomy)

A new experimental procedure for patients with outflow obstruction has been devised to reduce hypertrophy of the upper septum (and thereby outflow obstruction), without the need for open heart surgery, in severely symptomatic patients who no longer benefit from drugs (or pacing). This technique involves injecting a small amount of absolute alcohol solution (2-4 milliliters) into a minor (small) branch of the coronary artery that supplies the upper portion of the ventricular septum, thus destroying and thinning that part of the heart wall – and, in effect, producing a myocardial infarction and healed scar (i.e., "heart attack'). This technique is performed as part of a cardiac catheterization under local anesthetic. Although in relatively early stages of development, this technique may well represent a useful addition to the nonsurgical therapies available to patients with severe HCM symptoms.

The operative mortality for the ablation procedure and for myectomy surgery is similar in experienced centers. At present, the application of alcohol septal ablation to HCM patients remains a somewhat controversial issue with some interventional cardiologists advocating it with great enthusiasm and others suggesting restraint until the long-term consequences of the procedure can be assessed more completely. Also, there is concern that ablations are being performed with increasing frequency by cardiologists who are new to this technique, and possibly in some patients with less symptoms than are usually evidenced in the traditional surgical candidate. It should be emphasized that alcohol ablation is a procedure intended to be a potential *alternative to surgery,* and unless a patient clearly meets the criteria for the myotomy-myectomy operation they would not be candidates for ablation.

Of particular note, alcohol septal ablation leaves patients with a heart scar, which theoretically may predispose them to important arrhythmias later in life (unlike myotomy-myectomy, which leaves no such scar). For this reason, at the present time, we do not recommend septal ablation to young patients (and certainly not to children). Indeed, some referral institutions (such as the Cleveland Clinic) perform alcohol septal ablation only in operative candidates who otherwise are not optimal subjects for surgery, either because of associated medical conditions, strong patient preference against operation, or advanced age (70 years or older). Therefore, alcohol septal ablation, at present, is not regarded by most HCM physicians as either a cure or a primary treatment strategy for HCM, but rather as a potentially useful addition to the available treatment strategies for selected patients.

Pacemakers

Pacemakers have been used in HCM for several reasons. Occasionally, when the normal electrical signal fails to traverse the ventricles, either because of sinus node failure or heart block, implantation of a pacemaker is appropriate and necessary. This involves placing a small box containing a battery in the chest under the skin and passing fine wires through the veins to the heart in order to deliver the necessary signals so that the heart is automatically paced.

Over the past 8 years, many severely symptomatic patients with HCM and obstruction have received dual-chamber pacemakers for the purpose of relieving symptoms and outflow obstruction, as a treatment alternative to the septal myotomy-myectomy operation. Pacing can reduce the degree of obstruction in many patients but this is usually much less than achieved with operation. In addition, much of the symptom improvement perceived by many patients is probably due to a *placebo effect,* rather than real change in the disease state. It is essential to keep in mind that the most important issue in the treatment of any patient with HCM is whether an intervention (including pacing) improves symptoms and quality of life, and not its precise effect on the degree of obstruction. Certainly, pacemakers should not be regarded as a primary treatment for most patients with HCM, and the selection of which particular patients are likely to benefit from pacing is most important. At present, it appears that older patients with HCM (older than age 65) show the most convincing, positive effects from pacing.

One center has, in the past, recommended pacemakers for young children without symptoms to *prevent* the development of HCM. However, there is no reason to believe that a pacemaker can prevent a powerful genetic disease such as HCM from forming, progressing, or causing sudden death; furthermore, such an approach unnecessarily makes young children dependent on the pacemaker (and subject to pacemaker complications) for life. The Hypertrophic Cardiomyopathy Association (HCMA) and virtually all experts in the field do not recommend this treatment concept or strategy.

Heart Transplantation

For a small minority of HCM patients, heart transplantation may be recommended when there is severe disability and limiting symptoms, and marked impairment in the pumping action of the ventricles with enlargement of the heart chambers and thinning of the wall, which become unresponsive to other treatment. This facet of HCM is often referred to as the "end-stage" (or "dilated" or "burned-out" phase) and is the only generally accepted indication for heart transplantation within the disease spectrum of HCM. The end-stage ultimately affects only about 5-10% of patients. Spontaneously, and without a prior clinical event, the heart undergoes anatomic and functional changes that result in a form of heart failure more reminiscent of other heart diseases with greatly enlarged chambers (such as the dilated form of cardiomyopathy). As a result, the treatment for this type of heart failure clearly differs from that usually employed in HCM.

Of note, the end-stage phase represents an instance in the natural history of HCM during which there is considerable and spontaneous decrease in the thickness of the left ventricular wall, associated with an unfavorable clinical course (due to widespread scarring of the heart muscle). Therefore, the goal of curing HCM by reducing wall thickness (as has been suggested in one study with pacing) does not appear to be a realistic or a reasonably achievable objective for the treatment of this disease.

It is evident from this discussion that HCM is not a homogeneous disease and, certainly, that concept applies directly to treatment options. The disease spectrum of HCM is diagrammed in Figure 21.

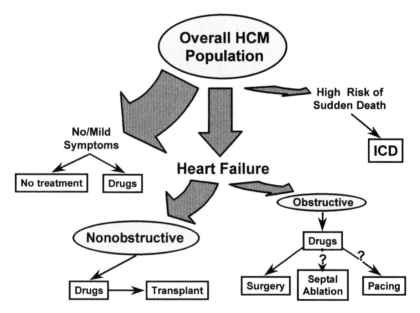

Figure 21. *Depiction of the very broad overall HCM disease spectrum.* Note, in particular, that many patients develop no or only mild symptoms, do not necessarily require treatment, and may achieve normal longevity in statistical terms. ICD = implantable cardioverter-defibrillator.

Is a Cure Available?

HCM as a Chronic Disease

Patients often ask whether there is a known cure for HCM. Strickly speaking, a cure for this disease is not available, i.e., if "cure" means the complete elimination of the disease process. Therefore, HCM must be regarded, at present, as a chronic disease. However, it is also very important to emphasize that HCM is not only compatible with normal longevity (with little or no disability and even without major treatment interventions), but its more serious complications can often be managed and controlled with drugs or implantable devices.

Therefore, HCM does not necessarily shorten life or have substantial impact on the quality of life. For example, in patients judged to be at high risk for sudden death, an ICD could be protective from such an event. For that individual patient, there may not be other risks related to the disease and, therefore, the ICD could possibly be regarded selectively as an HCM "cure." It is unlikely that, in the foreseeable future, gene therapy will ever be a workable or practical approach for HCM. Reducing wall thickening and hypertrophy (i.e., normalizing the heart structure) by drugs or other means is not a reasonable goal in HCM and, in fact, has never been shown to be possible.

Gene Therapy

Patients often inquire about the possibility of an HCM cure through gene therapy (in which "bad" genes are replaced by "good" or "normal" genes delivered directly into the body by a variety of methods), given the tremendous visibility, via the news media, of gene therapy and the human genome project. Conceptually, however, gene therapy will be a very difficult process in a disease genetically transmitted as autosomal dominant (such as is HCM). Standard models for which gene therapy has been proposed are other types of genetic diseases known as *recessive*. At present, gene therapy does not seem practical or largely applicable to HCM since the notion of introducing enough "good genes" to make all cells normal is regarded by molecular scientists as particularly daunting. Furthermore, gene therapy would not be without risk to the patient, raising ethical issues and great consternation as to which patients could or should be treated in this way. It should be kept in mind that a large proportion of patients with HCM experience a relatively benign course and can achieve normal life expectancy without such heroic interventions. Therefore, in purely theoretical terms, gene therapy would have to be confined to particularly high-risk patients and families, and even then probably in very young patients in whom hypertrophy has not yet become fully established. It is evident that the selection of HCM patients for gene therapy could be as complex as the treatment itself.

Family Screening

The majority of patients with HCM have at least one other affected relative, i.e., usually a parent, brother, sister, or child. When an individual is diagnosed as having HCM, all close relatives should be afforded the option of screening for the disease with an echocardiogram. It is important to remember that such a family evaluation is potentially important because HCM may be present, but not associated with any symptoms. A standard noninvasive outpatient evaluation includes a personal and family history, physical examination, ECG, and echocardiogram.

The standard and principal diagnostic test for the clinical diagnosis of HCM is the two-dimensional echocardiogram (with Doppler imaging). Laboratory DNA genotyping (using 10 cc of blood) theoretically would be the most definitive approach to diagnosis (i.e., by identification of a mutant gene). However, such laboratory techniques are expensive, laborious, not routinely available, and also do not guarantee a positive answer since all the genes that cause HCM are not yet known. Genetic testing is presently confined to a very small number of research laboratories that work on highly selected families, largely for research purposes. Hence, family screening for HCM is best carried out as it has been for many years – with the two-dimensional echocardiogram and ECG, often performed more than once in growing children from families with HCM.

The purpose of echocardiography, which is noninvasive and painless (and has an overall cost in the U.S. of about $600), is to identify what clinicians refer to as the ***phenotype*** or overt expression of HCM, i.e., the thickening of the left ventricular wall. It is important to keep in mind the important distinction that, while the mutant gene is present from birth, wall thickening usually develops later. Sometimes, HCM is referred to as a "congenital" disease (present from birth), but it is really only the genetic abnormality that is present from conception. This, of course, raises the question of when HCM becomes a "disease"– at birth, when the mutant gene is present, or when the heart wall becomes thick, or when symptoms occur. At present, this issue of nomenclature is unresolved.

The heart wall thickening is not usually evident before age 10 and is most likely to be detected in the adolescent years. Wall thickness usually increases as the child progresses through puberty with accelerated body growth and maturation (ages 12 to 16). Indeed, if wall thickening in an HCM family member becomes evident on the echocardiogram during adolescence, and cannot be explained in any another way (such as by long-term and intense athletic training or as other forms of heart disease), then it may be assumed to represent a mutant gene responsible for HCM. The changes in thickness with growth can be abrupt and striking and, therefore, the appearance of the heart can be altered completely during adolescence, often changing from completely normal to very thick. Experts believe these changes in hypertrophy, while often alarming in appearance to the family (and even some physicians), nevertheless represent the *normal pattern* in HCM (dictated by the DNA code) by which the heart reaches its mature form in this genetic disease. Therefore, the rapid heart growth (i.e., left ventricular wall thickening) commonly seen in teenagers does not necessarily represent deterioration, an alarming clinical sign, nor a warning of imminent danger. Furthermore, once hypertrophy is in place in mature adults, there is no evidence that it will increase further with aging. Therefore, the fear of many patients that their heart will continue to thicken through life, ultimately resulting in a catastrophic event, is completely unfounded. In fact, there is some evidence that wall thickness might decrease very slightly with advancing age in adults.

Based on the available evidence, we believe that (with some exceptions), if the hypertrophy is not present on the echocardiogram by the time full growth and maturation is achieved (about age 17-19 years), then it is unlikely to appear later. Recent research has shown that this rule is not invariably true, and some family members with particular mutant genes may not express their hypertrophy until much later in life. However, to date, only a very few genetically affected individuals have been documented to develop hypertrophy for the first time after age 30. Therefore, if an individual within an HCM family is "echo-negative" by the time adulthood begins, then there is a high likelihood (estimated at 90% or more) of not being affected by the mutant gene present in that family. Of course, if a family has been successfully genotyped in the laboratory (i.e., the family HCM gene has been found), then all the aforementioned uncertainty can be eliminated since it is relatively easy in such a circumstance to determine which relatives are affected by the family mutation.

When should echocardiograms be performed routinely in children within families with HCM? Screening echocardiograms before the age of 10 or 12 are optional since echocardiograms are rarely positive at that time, even in the presence of an HCM gene mutation, and recognition of the disease at this age does not usually necessitate treatment. An exception to this in which echocardiograms are obligatory at young ages would be in selected families with multiple occurrences of premature death due to HCM; early identification of high-risk individuals would be advantageous in terms of permitting potential preventive measures for sudden death. An echocardiogram is also recommended for young family members who are trained, competitive athletes, since

HCM is the most important cause of sudden death during sports in young people; to reduce that risk, the presence of HCM on an echocardiogram is a reason for disqualification from intense training and competition. In general, we recommend serial echocardiograms about every 18 months throughout adolescence or until the echocardiogram "converts" from normal to abnormal.

Strangely enough, the standard ECG may be abnormal in a genetically affected child long *before* the echocardiogram changes from normal to abnormal. For this reason, the ECG can also be useful as a screening test, even though it only records surface electrical signals and does not provide a direct image of heart structure (as does the echocardiogram). Of note, a small number of adults in HCM families with certain mutant genes may show no clinical evidence of HCM (i.e., normal echocardiogram and ECG, and also no symptoms); these individuals may nevertheless pass the HCM gene on to the next generation. This circumstance is, however, quite rare and is limited to certain mutations; very few patients with normal echocardiograms after age 21 have later converted to thickened hearts.

What About
Having Children? Pregnancy and Delivery

Even if a child inherits the abnormal HCM gene, the degree to which he or she will be affected by the *disease* is to a large extent unpredictable. There is no consistently reliable method for predicting precisely how severe HCM might be in an offspring and, in fact, there is considerable variability in this regard, even within families. A mildly affected parent can have a severely affected child, or vice versa. Alternatively, an entire family may have "benign" disease, while (albeit uncommon) other families have "malignant" forms of HCM in which several relatives die prematurely or have severe disease and disability. Therefore, the decision whether to have children must be an individual choice, based on all these considerations including the particular expression of the disease in the family.

For the vast majority of women with HCM, pregnancy and vaginal delivery poses no added risk and is well-tolerated and safe. However, for the rare female HCM patient with severe symptoms or important arrhythmias, pregnancy could carry additional risk, and Cesarean section may be considered selectively to achieve some control over the medical circumstances. Obviously, such women should have access to specialized high-risk obstetrical care. Maternal death (or infant death) due to HCM as a consequence of childbirth is virtually unknown and unreported.

Women may find that they develop symptoms for the first time during pregnancy, or that preexisting symptoms are intensified. Also, the issue of taking cardiac drugs around the time of conception or during pregnancy arises in many cases. Drugs such as beta-blockers and calcium channel blockers (such as verapamil) taken by the mother have access to the fetus, because they are capable of crossing the placental barrier, and could in theory damage the baby. There is little direct evidence, however, of damage to the fetus due to the administration of these drugs to the mother. Nevertheless, it is best to be cautious, if possible, and to avoid all drugs during pregnancy (certainly in the first trimester). For all these reasons, it is prudent for patients with HCM to plan their pregnancy in advance, and to discuss all pertinent medical issues at an early stage with a cardiologist and an obstetrician. Also, it may be best to avoid epidural anesthesia at delivery (particularly in women with gradients), as this may cause an excessive fall in blood pressure and could increase obstruction.

Routine Medical Care

Patients with HCM should be seen regularly by a cardiologist near their home even if they are stable and do not develop new complaints. Clinic visits on an annual basis seem to work out the best. Many patients complain that their cardiologist openly expresses inexperience with HCM. This, of course, is not an uncommon occurrence because of the rarity of HCM in the general population, as well as in cardiological practice. Some patients alleviate this frustration by electing to be seen concurrently by one of several HCM consultants, i.e., cardiologists with a special interest and expertise in HCM. Please contact the HCMA for names of HCM experts (phone: 973-983-7429; fax: 973-983-7439; e-mail: support@hcma-heart.com). We chose not to publish such a list of cardiologists and surgeons, which would likely become outdated with time. It is also a good idea for a primary care physician (i.e., a general practitioner or internist) to be involved in the care of an HCM patient. Of course, for those patients who are symptomatic and require treatment, more frequent follow-up may be required with a cardiologist or another specialist such as an electrophysiologist (e.g., if a defibrillator is implanted). Generally, if the patient is stable and new issues do not arise, medical visits that occur no more frequently than at 1-year intervals (with echocardiogram, ECG, and Holter assessments) are standard.

General Lifestyle Advice

Diet

Sensible eating habits are encouraged to maintain body weight within the normal range for height and age. If an individual is overweight, this places extra unnecessary strain on the heart in HCM, as it would for any cardiac condition. Attention should also be paid to cholesterol levels, as would be advised for any patient. However, it should be emphasized that elevated cholesterol is a risk factor for coronary artery disease, and not specifically for HCM. No special diet or vitamin supplementation is required for HCM. A rapid increase in weight is likely to be due to fluid retention, and the patient's physician should be notified. Excessive salt intake should be avoided, but unless heart failure is in its advanced stages, low salt diets are not usually advised.

Exercise

For most patients, HCM will not interfere importantly with lifestyle. Some individuals may have symptoms related to exertion and find that they cannot undertake as much physical work or recreation as other people their age. Under these circumstances, medical advice should be sought before undertaking physically demanding activities. Patients with HCM and symptoms such as shortness of breath, chest pain, or lightheadedness during activity (even if mild) should not extend themselves into physical activities that have the effect of inducing or accentuating symptoms. Such symptoms are an indication or warning that heart function has been impaired. It is best to consider the axiom: have a good measure of respect for your disease (in this case, HCM). Most experts believe that individuals with HCM should not participate in competitive sports or other particularly strenuous physical activities. This recommendation is based on the observation that intense physical exertion appears to predispose some susceptible individuals with HCM (and also with other forms of heart disease) to sudden death.

Nevertheless, after these considerations are taken into account, it is a reasonable expectation that most affected individuals with HCM will be able to adopt a normal or near-normal lifestyle, including certain normal recreational activities. HCM patients should seek the advice of their cardiologist as to the specific type of recreational exercise program that should be undertaken.

Exercise programs for patients with HCM should not be confused with participation in competitive sports or even certain intense recreational athletic activities. HCM patients are not compelled to lead a completely sedentary lifestyle. For example, walking and toning (not using free weights) are two generally acceptable forms of exercise. However, all exercise programs should be initiated with some caution. The patient may want to inquire with the physician about entering a cardiac rehabilitation program where he/she will be monitored while performing exercises that promote good general health. These programs also provide the security of assistance from a medical team, should a problem arise.

In many families, participation in sports has been a tradition, and/or played a very large role in daily life. These activities may have, in fact, become a major focus and important part of the social life of not only the child, but of the entire family. It will be difficult for a child (regardless of age), after receiving a diagnosis of HCM, to understand that he/she can no longer participate in competitive sports. When a diagnosis of HCM is made in a committed athlete, it is perhaps more devastating than the same diagnosis in a nonathletic child. Children who are experienced athletes will require assistance to redirect their time to other activities (which may include certain recreational sports). Therefore, it is important to encourage the child to maintain existing relationships with athletic friends, but at the same time extend their network of friends to those who participate in other activities. At the same time, it will also be difficult for parents, who have developed friends and a social circle connected to these sporting events, to no longer be able to participate. Some parents can find it just as difficult dealing with this loss as does the child. Finding a new family activity in which new friends and traditions can be developed may be important. This transition in lifestyle may be difficult, and professional counseling may be of assistance during this time.

Keep in mind that habitual vigorous exercise has many benefits in middle-aged and older individuals for preventing the adverse consequences of coronary artery disease; however, this is a much different situation than in HCM.

Alcohol

Patients with HCM should avoid excessive consumption of alcohol because of its potentially adverse effects on heart muscle. Also, one study has shown that outflow obstruction may actually increase after very small amounts of alcohol, probably due to the dilatation of blood vessels that is produced by the drug. On the other hand, the modest daily consumption of beer or wine is certainly acceptable.

Viagra

Sudden death and other adverse consequences with the use of Viagra (sildenafil citrate) have been reported in a small minority of patients with symptomatic coronary artery disease. However, because HCM is uncommon, there are no data governing side effects of Viagra in HCM. Nevertheless, there are important theoretical reasons to avoid Viagra if HCM is present. Because this drug dilates arterial vessels it could increase obstruction and be dangerous to HCM patients. We believe, therefore, that HCM patients should avoid using Viagra.

Flu Vaccination

This may be recommended by the physician to prevent influenza, particularly in very young and elderly individuals. The presence of HCM does not exclude this treatment, although the patient (or parents, in the case of young children) should be aware that there are occasional side effects from the vaccine (which also may not provide absolute protection against infection).

Other Restrictions

- *Acute severe loss of blood or body fluid:* hemorrhage, diarrhea, vomiting, if excessive, can lead to unfavorable consequences such as increased obstruction.
- *Prolonged standing in hot baths or showers:* may predispose to fainting or near-fainting.
- *During anesthesia (including an epidural at the time of child-birth):* special attention is required to avoid a sudden drop in blood pressure. There have been a few reports suggesting an increased risk associated with epidural anesthesia; this procedure should probably be avoided in HCM patients, particularly in the presence of outflow obstruction.
- *Prolonged and extreme hot and cold conditions:* can predispose to unfavorable consequences such as arrhythmias.

Psychological Adjustment to HCM

The effect of chronic illness on a patient and family is similar to that of other emotional trauma, but with certain differences. Chronic diseases produce the feelings of fear, grief, and loss that are essentially unending. A chronic illness such as HCM (which incorporates a risk for sudden cardiac death in some individuals) presents patients and their family with a lack of predictability that may make adjustment to daily life more difficult. There is the constant living with the unknown and an acute sense of lack of control over events. This circumstance may be perceived as "living with a sword over one's head." In contrast, in most other instances of loss, as tragic as they may be, there is at least a finality that must be accepted; shock and denial give way to acceptance and adaptation.

The following scenario can be imagined. Someone says, "Carry this beeper. One day it may go off and you must respond immediately and correctly. It will be the most important moment of your life. It could go off next week, next year, or 10 years from now...but be ready." This somewhat analogous situation will obviously create chronic anxiety and anger in patients, and in their family and friends as well, and is essentially what happens with a disease such as HCM. A medical condition can itself become an anxiety state characterized by preoccupation and hyperalertness and can paralyze the patient's adjustment to daily life activities. Eventually, depression can result when the constant state of anxiety (and often a sense of hopelessness) gradually wears down the patient's reserves. There is often a profound sense of unfairness ("how and why did this happen to me") and lack of control over the situation, but also the realization that life is imperfect. The trauma created by chronic diseases can also result in reprioritization of life goals and values, which may represent a positive consequence of an otherwise negative situation.

A disruption of the family "homeostasis" may result, and the roles that members have played for years can be thrown into disarray. There may also be substantial guilt involved in HCM families, i.e., for having transmitted the disease to children. This may relate to the dilemma faced by many patients, of deciding to have children (and to take the chance of transmitting the mutant gene). Genetic counseling is an important component of treatment for HCM, as it may help to answer such difficult and delicate questions for patients. Certainly, in many families there is not an absolutely correct answer to such decisions, as a number of considerations may be involved, including variability in the clinical expression of the gene defect within and between families. Furthermore, and most importantly, for the majority of patients with

HCM it is unrealistic to live in terror of the possibility of deterioration and premature death, since it is now evident that this disease often has a benign course with normal longevity.

Chronic diseases such as HCM present a series of dilemmas and a continuum of choices for patients. As a goal, we recommend achieving a psychological state somewhere in between the following extremes:

- From ignoring symptoms and "toughing it out"—to overreacting to symptoms;
- From looking for miracle cures (and possibly doing harm) – to unwisely trusting everything a physician relates;
- From keeping the illness a secret, and risking deception – to discussing it too openly, and risking the perception of self-pity;
- From asking for help, and risking becoming a burden – to holding steadfast to independence, and risking isolation;
- From insisting that family and friends behave as if everything is normal, and denying them the expression and release of feelings – to allowing family and friends to be overprotective, at the risk of becoming dependent and childlike;
- From straining the body to its physical limits, and risking self harm – to "playing it safe" and becoming an invalid;
- From living in fear of degeneration and death, and risking immobilization – to regarding each day as a special and pristine dispensation;
- From insisting on controlling life at the risk of frustration – to "going with the flow," and risking passivity;
- From being angry at fate, and risking bitterness – to focusing only on blessings, and risking self-delusion.

Fortunately, it is a characteristic of human beings that strength can be drawn from adversity. This can be facilitated by mutual support between patients and their families, and by interaction among patients afflicted with the same disease. This process includes acknowledging "what could have been," accepting and adapting to the reality of the given situation, and finding ways to make life meaningful despite a chronic illness. It is also important that as many immediate and extended family members as possible participate in this "renewal." In addition, the family that has been traumatized by chronic illness (in this case, by HCM) will thereby be able to take collective pride in this newfound strength.

Finally, patients should refrain from seeking miracle solutions; they should be cautious and discriminating about accepting seemingly unrealistic, dramatic predictions related to "cures," regardless of the source. Perhaps, it is best to regard treatment advances in HCM in the context of *controlling* the disease, rather than as cures in absolute terms.

Support and Advocacy Groups

"Support groups" take a variety of forms, including the family unit and close friends. As individuals, however, we often find the need to discuss unique issues and problems, or find answers to complex questions that our family or friends may not be able to provide.

Such as been the rationale for support or advocacy groups focused on specific (often uncommon) medical conditions. Previously, such advocacy groups were largely located in a particular geographical area or community for the purpose of meeting to discuss common problems and sharing insights. This format allowed each person to seek the support of others affected by the same life circumstances they had experienced.

Many physicians understand the need for and benefits of support groups. Moreover, recent studies have proven that a positive attitude has a direct relationship to a patient's quality of life. Support groups offer patients and families the information, support, and education needed to cope more effectively with their medical condition. In addition to a better quality of life for the patient, the entire family will benefit from a clearer understanding of the condition (which in some cases represents a family disease). The understanding gained from the support group may also help the patient communicate more effectively with his/her physician. More recently, the advent of the Internet has created an inexpensive and instantaneous free-flow of information and contact between interested parties, creating online support groups independent of geography or even international boundaries. This easier and more efficient dissemination of information has made a marked difference for patients with uncommon diseases, such as HCM.

The Hypertrophic Cardiomyopathy Association (HCMA) was founded in 1996 by Lisa Salberg in the memory of her sister, Lori Anne Flanigan, who died suddenly of HCM. It was the aspiration of the founder to help others with HCM to have a clearer understanding of their disease, as well as access to all available treatment options.

Indeed, one of the key elements of the HCMA is to provide appropriate and accurate information to the patient (who is often confused about his/her disease) through direct exposure to the medical literature or expert clinicians. Traditionally, patients with HCM become confused by the scientific literature – which is often characterized by exaggerated pessimism – or by a limited familiarity with HCM on the part of their local physicians. However, the technological advance of the Internet has changed that situation by affording: (1) enhanced communication, and specifically, by offering HCM patients the opportunity to be more appropriately informed regarding the nature and implications of their disease; (2) increased contact among patients; and (3) access to experts in HCM. In addition, all of the improvements in the access to information for the patient may be supplemented by more traditional "in-person" support meetings on a regional basis.

The following are the specific goals and objectives of the HCMA:

- To develop and maintain a network of support for people with HCM, their families, and the medical community;
- To provide education about the symptoms, risks, and treatment options to those living with HCM, as well as to those delivering professional care to HCM patients;
- To raise awareness regarding protection against sudden death;
- To develop and maintain a network of health care providers educated in the diagnosis and treatment of HCM;
- To promote additional research on HCM and its treatment, and to provide easy access to this information.

The HCMA provides a vast number of services to its membership including, but not limited to:

- Regionally located, person-to-person meetings
- Emotional support to individual patients and families with HCM
- Information about, and access to, medical providers
- Education to patients, medical practitioners, and community advocacy groups
- Internet-based access including bulletin board information
- International contacts to further the interest of its members

The HCMA also provides individual and confidential support for matters related to:

- Concerns regarding a recent diagnosis
- Questions about "centers of excellence" in the field of HCM
- Information on the condition and treatment options
- Support to families who may have lost a loved one to HCM
- Access to other HCM patients with whom they share a unique bond

The HCMA provides those with HCM (or their family members) with the ability to make direct contact with other HCM patients. After a "rare" genetic disorder has been diagnosed, access to others with the same problem provides a sense of belonging and the assurance that the patient "is not alone."

How to Contact Other HCM Support Groups

Cardiomyopathy Association
40 The Metro Centre
Tolpits Lane
Watford, Herts WD1 8SB
United Kingdom

Phone: (44) 1923-249977
Fax: (44) 1923-249987
www.cardiomyopathy.org

The Hypertrophic Cardiomyopathy
   Association of Canada
305-4625 Varsity Drive, Suite 65
N.W. Calgary, AB T3A OZ9
Canada

Phone: 403-289-7834
www.hcmacc.com

Cardiomyopathy Association of
   Australia, Ltd.
26 Clanalpine Street
Mosman, NSW 2088
Australia

Phone: (61) 3 9439 1133

The Montgomery Foundation
   Robert Montgomery, MD, PhD, and
   Meg Montgomery
Primarily for dilated cardiomyopathy

Phone: 410-254-6370
Fax: 410-254-6379
rmonty@welchlink.welch.jhu.edu

The Mended Hearts, Inc.
7272 Greenville Avenue
Dallas, TX 75231-4596
For those who have had cardiac surgery

Living With HCM: Other Considerations

Driving

A diagnosis of HCM should have no bearing on the patient's personal driving license and privileges. If symptoms of syncope (fainting) or near-syncope (near-fainting) have been experienced, the physician may advise the patient not to drive until these symptoms can be better controlled.

If the patient cannot walk long distances without symptoms such as shortness of breath, chest pain, or lightheadedness it is suggested that he/she apply for a handicapped parking permit. In many cases, this involves a simple form that can be obtained from the local motor vehicle office (and which must be signed by the doctor).

Patients who have implantable defibrillators should consult with their doctors regarding local regulations governing automobile driving with these devices. In several states, it is suggested that defibrillator patients should not drive for up to 6 months after the implant. The patient and the physician should discuss the individual situation and decide what is the best strategy.

To be qualified as a taxi or truck driver with a Commercial Drivers License (CDL), a complete physical examination is necessary. There is precedent, with a diagnosis of HCM, for denial of a CDL. However, there is also an appeals process, and with the evaluation of a cardiologist, it may be possible to eventually obtain a CDL. Reevaluation is required annually, and therefore a repetitive appeal process may be necessary. Therefore, we do not advise careers in this field for patients with HCM.

Traveling

Health concerns must be considered when planning a trip. It is important to remember to bring all medications and it is always a good idea to have a letter explaining the medical condition. In U.S. airports, assistance can be requested for transport to the gate; foreign airports vary greatly and the travel agent should be asked to make these arrangements. For those who are more symptomatic, it is critical to remember the importance of pacing oneself while on vacation, or fatigue may subsequently interfere with enjoyment. Calling ahead is a good idea to determine how far away attractions are, and, if necessary, to arrange for a motorized scooter or wheelchair. For example, major theme parks provide rental scooters and wheelchairs on site. If the trip is for business purposes, ample travel time should be allotted, to allow for rest before meetings.

Commercial airline travel itself (at the altitudes conventionally involved) poses no risk to HCM patients. Caution should be exercised in scheduling vacations or trips to remote destinations where the level of medical care is rudimentary and/or where specific knowledge of HCM may be virtually nonexistent. The same considerations apply to traveling on cruise ships, where the level of medical care may not be consistent and, in some instances, suboptimal for an individual with HCM. Those who have implantable defibrillators and who are planning trips may want to contact the electrophysiologist (or the device manufacturer) to identify the nearest suitable hospital to the vacation/business destination. Customer service phone numbers for device manufacturers are:

Medtronic   800-635-3525
Guidant   800-227-3422
St. Jude Medical   800-328-9634

Military Service

For those wishing to enter the Armed Forces. Careers in the military are not encouraged for those with HCM for a variety of reasons. However, anyone who desires to pursue this career path should be aware of the following. As a general guideline, the military will disqualify any person with "hypertrophy" or "dilatation" of the heart. If a person with HCM wishes to enter the military, there is an appeals process in which a petition can be made to the Service Waive Authorities for reevaluation. If a person has long-term disease stability, a waiver may be awarded. However, due to the variable nature of HCM, it is unlikely that such a waiver would be awarded. If the HCM diagnosis "slips by" at recruitment or service entry and is established later, that person will be removed from the military and possibly prosecuted for misrepresentation.

For those currently serving in the military. Many factors are evaluated by the military in determining whether a person with any newly discovered medical condition may remain in active service. Several issues will be considered in the case of a diagnosis of HCM including (but not limited to) length of service, job assignment, and qualifications. If it occurs early in a person's career, it is unlikely that the military will retain that person, who may then wish to apply for military disability. Military disability will pay a portion of wages, but is not the same as Social Security Disability. The intent of military disability is, in most cases, to return the person to the civilian world where employment will be available. If the person already has an extensive military career, it is likely that an assessment of the specific job functions can be requested. If that person is "fit for duty" they may remain in their assignment. If not, a new position and a revised training program may be provided. However, with increasing frequency, the military is attempting to ensure – for matters of public safety, but also in the best interests of soldiers with a disease such as HCM – that recruits are World Wide Qualified. This means that that person must be able to work anywhere the military might send them, without consideration for the availability of specific or specialized medical treatment. For example, if a person has an ICD, and is stationed in a remote area, would the military be able to provide the care necessary to ensure that person's health and well-being?

The Americans with Disabilities Act does not provide protection for those in the U.S. military. Those who live outside the U.S. should check with local military recruitment centers to inquire as to the specific country's military guidelines.

Social Security Benefits

Those in the U.S who have severe limitations in daily life functions because of HCM may be eligible for Social Security Disability Insurance (SSDI) coverage. However, a diagnosis of HCM is not itself sufficient to claim disability under SSDI. The Social Security Administration defines "disability" as the inability to do any kind of work for which the person is suited and trained; the disability is expected to last for a least 1 year.

SSDI benefits can be received at any age. If SSDI benefits are received at age 65, that amount will become the retirement benefit. Dependents may be eligible for additional Social Security insurance benefits if the household income is low enough to create financial need. Dependents include:

- Unmarried children, including stepchildren, adopted children, or in some cases, grandchildren, under the age of 18 (or 19 if still a full-time high school student).
- Unmarried children, 18 or older, if the disability occurred before the age of 22.
- A spouse, if 62 or older, or any age if he or she is caring for a child who is under 16 or disabled, and also receiving disability checks.
- A disabled widow or widower 50 years or older. The disability must have occurred before, or within 7 years after (the HCM patient's), death.
- A disabled ex-wife or ex-husband who is 50 years or older, if the marriage lasted at least 10 years.

The local Social Security office will send applications to the state's Disability Determination Service (DDS) office. A team consisting of a physician (or psychologist) and a disability evaluation specialist will consider all facts and decide if the applicant is "disabled" by Social Security's definition. The team of professionals is asked to determine whether you can perform work-related activities such as walking, sitting, lifting, and carrying.

If the claim is denied, there are four levels of appeal available. As this is a complicated process, many persons choose to have an attorney represent them. For more information on Social Security, direct calls can be made to 800-772-1213.

Family and Medical Leave Act

The Family and Medical Leave Act (FMLA) became effective in 1993. The purpose of the Act is to help balance the demands of the workplace with the needs of families by allowing eligible employees to take up to 12 weeks of unpaid, job-protected leave (during any 12-month period) for specific family emergencies such as serious illness or the birth of a child. Employers who have 50 or more employees working 20 or more weeks in the current or preceding calendar year and who are engaged in commerce are covered, as well as public agencies (including governmental agencies and schools). To be eligible, an employee must have worked:

1. For a covered employer at least 12 months.
2. At least 1,250 hours during the past 12 months; and at a location where at least 50 other employees are living within 75 miles of the workplace.

Life Insurance

While the diagnosis of HCM will not always leave you "uninsurable," it may nevertheless result in very high premiums. You must disclose all medical information to the insurance company. With this in mind, it may be a wise idea to purchase coverage *prior to* being screened for HCM. If you have already been diagnosed with HCM, you can purchase coverage from a number of "assigned risk" carriers. A better idea is to maximize any group insurance your employer, credit card company, or civic organization may offer.

Coverage for children may be taken as a "rider" on an existing adult policy. These provisions are in most cases "non-medical,'" which means that no medical questions are asked regarding the child. Many "riders" can be converted to a separate policy at age 18, and at as much as five times the original value. This is a good way to ensure coverage for the child into adulthood.

Implantable Defibrillators

Many patients and their families have questions about the potential interaction between an automatic ICD and electromagnetic fields in the environment. First, it is important to understand the nature of an elecromagnetic field. Simply stated, it is an invisible line of force resulting from the use of electricity, such as devices plugged into an outlet or operated by a battery.

Most of the equipment and appliances we come into contact with on a daily basis will not effect an ICD. It is generally a good idea, however, for patients to keep their distance from devices that generate large amounts of electromagnetic interference such as welding instruments and large electrical generators. Nevertheless, ICD recipients should be able to safely operate most household appliances, tools, and machines that are properly grounded and in good repair. Examples of electrical equipment that do not cause interference include:

- Microwave ovens
- Televisions, AM/FM radios, VCRs
- Tabletop appliances such as electric toasters, blenders, knives, and can openers
- Handheld devices such as shavers and hair dryers
- Electric blankets and heating pads
- Major appliances including washers, dryers, and electric stoves
- Personal computers, photocopiers, and electric typewriters
- Light industrial equipment such as drills and table saws (not including battery-powered tools)

ICDs are sensitive to particularly strong electrical or magnetic fields, which have the potential to deactivate some devices, although this occurs only on very rare occasions. In some cases, an ICD may emit a sound if it is too close to a magnetic field. If this happens, it is important to move away from the object and location immediately.

The potential sources of strong electrical and magnetic fields listed below should be kept at least 12 inches (30 centimeters) away from an ICD pulse generator:

- Stereo speakers from large systems, transistor radios, "boom boxes," or similar instruments
- Strong magnets
- Magnetic wands used by airport security and in other circumstances
- Industrial equipment such as power generators and welding instruments
- Battery-powered cordless power tools such as screwdrivers, drills, etc.

It is important to avoid leaning over an engine that is running, because alternators frequently emit magnetic fields. ICD pulse generators may also be sensitive to anti-theft systems, also called electronic article surveillance (EAS) systems, which are frequently found in stores and public libraries. These systems, which typically consist of one or two columns placed near entrances and exists, are sometimes hidden or camouflaged so as to be unobtrusive. An ICD will not be affected by such systems while walking at a normal pace through the public entrances and exits. However, lingering in an EAS field may adversely affect an ICD.

Airport security alarm systems (both the portals through which a person walks or the handheld wand used by security personnel) use magnetic fields for the purpose of detecting metal. The security portals, or archways, will not harm the device, but it is prudent to walk through at a normal pace and not linger near them. However, the handheld wand *could deactivate some ICD devices* if held directly over the pulse generator for a relatively short period of time. For this reason, ICD identification and security cards should be shown to airport security personnel, and patients are encouraged to request an alternative search performed by hand. If security personnel insist on using the wand, the procedure should be performed quickly, and the wand should not linger over the device.

Some cellular phones, if placed closer than 6 inches (15 centimeters) to the pulse generator, could adversely affect the mechanism by which an ICD device senses arrhythmias. It is important to note that this potential effect is temporary, and that moving the phone away from the device will restore proper function of the ICD system. Therefore, a few precautions will reduce the chance of any interaction. It is advisable to keep the cellular phone at least 6 inches (15 centimeters) away from an ICD pulse generator. If the phone transmits more than 3 watts of power, increase that minimum distance to 12 inches (30 centimeters). Always keep the cellular phone on the opposite side of the body from the ICD pulse generator. Do not carry a cellular phone in a breast pocket or on a belt if that places the phone within 6 inches (15 centimeters) of the pulse generator.

Please note that such precautions need *not* apply to household cordless phones because such instruments transmit signals with less energy and will not interfere with the ICD device.

Dental and Other Medical Procedures

Dental drills and cleaning equipment will not interfere with an ICD system. Patients with ICDs should be aware, however, that special precautions must be taken with the following procedures:

- Diathermy uses an electrical field to apply heat to body tissues. An ICD device could be affected by the electrical current used during this procedure.
- Electrocautery, a procedure that uses an electronic device to stop bleeding, should be used only when the ICD system is turned off.
- Magnetic resonance imaging (MRI; also called nuclear magnetic resonance [NMR]) is a diagnostic test that uses a strong electromagnetic field and creates high resolution images of the heart. These magnets can impair the ICD device. Patients who have ICDs should not enter hospital rooms marked "MRI."

What Research Is Being Conducted?

There are several active HCM research programs largely in the U.S., Canada, Europe, and Japan. Some of this research is aimed at identifying and characterizing the genetic mutations and other abnormalities responsible for the disease, and is being conducted in selected laboratories (in the U.S., primarily at Brigham and Women's Hospital, Harvard Medical School, Boston, MA, and also Baylor University Medical Center, Houston, TX). It is the view of many molecular biologists that knowledge of the basic genetic defect responsible for HCM in each patient will ultimately permit earlier, more definitive intervention, and more targeted and tailored treatment.

Additional efforts emphasize further definition and clarification of the diagnostic features and clinical course of HCM, as well as the development and application of novel treatment strategies. For example, introduction of the ICD for HCM has changed the course of the disease for many patients. However, as is true with many other uncommon diseases, relatively few clinical investigators are focusing their research interests on HCM. Consequently (and unfortunately), financial support for HCM research (particularly clinical investigation) is relatively sparse at present. Nevertheless, the ongoing research efforts related to HCM are regarded as vigorous, although the emphasis changes periodically. Patients and physicians are therefore encouraged to contact the HCMA for the most current information regarding HCM research.

The 27 Most Frequently
Asked Questions by Patients about HCM
(addressed to the HCMA)

1. *Did I catch HCM from an infection?*

No, HCM is a genetic disease. This means you were born with a mutation in a gene which causes HCM. You may not have had symptoms or known you had HCM, but nevertheless you were indeed born with it. However, what actually triggers the mutation itself to occur is unknown and environmental factors could conceivably play a role.

2. *I always have symptoms of dizziness and chest pain, and sometimes I am short of breath. I hate to bother my doctor, but when should I call him (her)?*

You should discuss your symptoms, in as much detail as appropriate, with your doctor. Ask what you should do if you feel you are in danger for any reason. You may be told to come to the office or go directly to an emergency room if your symptoms are more severe than usual. If you are in doubt, call your doctor or go to the emergency room.

3. *Should I have children?*

This cannot be a "yes" or "no" answer, but is largely a matter of individual choice. It is a very common question from both the male and female members of the HCMA. A child born to a parent with HCM has a statistical 50/50 chance of inheriting a mutant gene for HCM. It is important to remember that most people with HCM live normal lives with the necessity of little or no medical intervention. Therefore, genetic counselors rarely advise against having children, although in those families with multiple sudden deaths and particularly serious disease ("malignant HCM"), consideration should be given to not propagating the malignant mutant gene. Women with HCM can usually experience normal pregnancies, and there are no data to suggest that it is generally harmful to be pregnant with HCM. In some cases, a woman can remain on certain heart medications during the entire pregnancy (your obstetrician should be consulted about this). Delivery can occasionally convey some added risks in selected patients with HCM. Epidural anesthesia has been associated with a few reported deaths in Europe, and therefore, we suggest that you discuss this issue with your doctor well before delivery. If you choose to become pregnant you may also want to discuss breast feeding with your doctor to be sure your medications will not adversely affect the baby.

4. Can I exercise? Which types of activities should I participate in and which should I avoid?

Moderate exercise is fine. Walking, swimming, skating, golf, bowling, and yoga/Ti chi are examples of activities in which you may feel comfortable participating. Intensive sports or competitive situations, particularly those involving "burst" exertion (such as basketball) should be avoided. You should consult with your own doctor about the most appropriate recreational exercise program to ensure that you are not placing yourself at an added risk.

5. Will HCM affect my sex life?

HCM, as well as some medications used to treat the disease, can cause fatigue, so there may be a lack of energy rather than an absence of interest. Some medications, such as beta-blockers, can in fact cause impotence. In general, however, those with HCM should be able to enjoy a normal sex life.

6. Sometimes I think I am depressed. It is hard living with a chronic disease. What can I do to feel better?

Do not be afraid to discuss your feelings with your doctor. Depression can be a consequence of how you perceive your life situation, or possibly a side effect of some cardiac drugs. Therefore, you may need to change medications to help relieve your depression. If a drug reaction is not causing your depression, you may need to see a psychiatrist, psychologist, or another mental health clinician to discuss your feelings. Certainly, living with a chronic disease *is* difficult and you should not hesitate to seek help in dealing with the emotional component of the condition. In families where there has been a death related to HCM, and other family members also have HCM, family/group counseling may prove helpful.

7. Will my heart get bigger?

After reaching full maturity, normally by age 18-20 years, your heart growth usually stops. You may be aware of slight changes in measurements of the thickness of the left ventricular wall, but generally the thickness will remain about the same. There are extraordinary exceptions, but this rule covers about 90-95% of the relevant clinical situations.

8. I thought it was good to have big muscles, so what is wrong with a thick heart muscle?

Having "big" muscles may sound like a good thing to some. However, an abnormally thick heart muscle is not beneficial to your health, particularly if the thickening creates a situation in which the heart cannot properly fill with blood during the relaxation phase (diastole), such as may occur in HCM.

9. *I live in a remote area, the local hospital is very small, and I am afraid the medical staff will not know how to help me. What can I do to help them help me?*

Take a proactive role in your own health care. Stop by the local emergency room on a day you are feeling well and bring them information (such as this book). This will allow you the opportunity to speak to the staff when you are not in an emergency situation. By doing this, you will also provide those health care workers with the opportunity to read and research HCM so that they will be ready for you in case you need them.

10. *I get very tired after a big meal. Is this normal, or is it from HCM?*

This is a very common complaint among HCM patients. We suggest you eat smaller meals and try to avoid heavy foods. You will also want to avoid eating late at night. There is, in fact, some evidence that a heavy meal can accentuate outflow obstruction.

11. *Are there any other conditions that cause HCM? Or, can HCM cause any other conditions?*

There are syndromes that have been associated with HCM. Noonan's syndrome is one such condition that is associated with a thick heart muscle (but differs in its genetic basis from true HCM). There are also other syndromes (some in infants) that may mimic HCM in appearance, but are not really the same disease. HCM does not "cause" these other conditions.

12. *Is it usual to feel tired because of HCM?*

Yes, fatigue is probably the most common complaint we hear at the HCMA; however, it is a different symptom from shortness of breath with exertion. The basis for fatigue in HCM is not well understood.

13. *Can I drink caffeine and eat salt?*

You should consult with your doctor for your own specific dietary restrictions and needs. Caffeine can have adverse reactions in some people and cause a racing heart. If you are prone to arrhythmias, you may want to avoid caffeine products. Keep in mind that there is a substantial amount of caffeine in products other than coffee, such as cola drinks (including diet colas), tea, and chocolate. Salt (sodium) may be harmful to those with high blood pressure or heart failure.

14. How important is my cholesterol level?

Just because you have HCM does not mean you are at any less risk for other forms of cardiovascular disease. Some older people with HCM also have coronary artery disease (mostly over age 50). Therefore, it is always a good idea to maintain a "heart healthy" diet. HCM is not protective in any way against atherosclerosis.

15. Should I tell my cousins, aunts, uncles, or other blood relatives that I have been diagnosed with HCM?

Yes, although it may be difficult to talk about this, you are obligated to let your family know. All blood relatives should be screened for HCM (with echocardiography), particularly if there have been premature deaths due to heart disease in the family.

16. Why can't they just cut my heart "down to size"?

HCM is a complex disease and, even if this were possible, normalizing the heart structure would not necessarily be the answer to the overall problem. It would be scientifically and medically untenable to remove enough abnormal muscle by surgery or any means. Also, even portions of the heart wall with normal thickness may be abnormal in terms of function. Patients with outflow obstruction can have surgical procedures to rectify that problem. Even then only a small amount of muscle is removed by the surgeon (i.e., 3–6 grams); the usual overall heart weight is about 500 grams.

17. Can I drink alcohol?

There are little data on alcohol consumption in HCM, but moderation is advised. Alcohol could have a depressant effect on the heart muscle. Also, consumption of even a small amount of alcohol has been shown to raise the gradient by acting as a stimulant.

18. What effect will marijuana have on someone with HCM?

There is no direct evidence related to the effect of marijuana on HCM. Nevertheless, it is the conservative and prudent position of the HCMA that marijuana should be avoided as there are no data one way or the other to say what possible complications could arise from interactions between the drug and disease.

19. What effect will the use of cocaine, heroin, or ecstasy have on someone with HCM?

Although their precise effect on HCM is not known with certainty, the use of these types of "recreational" drugs could prove to be adverse in someone with a complex disease such as HCM, and should be avoided.

20. Can I become a pilot?

In the U.S., a commercial pilot must pass a physical examination annually for the Federal Aviation Administration. At present, in the U.S., it is possible to obtain a third-class (private aircraft) license with HCM, although a first class commercial license may be associated with difficulties for most individuals with HCM.

21. Are there any occupations I should avoid?

You may want to avoid occupations that predominantly require physical labor. In some patients, intense physical activity (occupational or recreational) could prove detrimental. In addition, if you have an implanted device (pacemaker/defibrillator) you will need to avoid certain occupations such as those requiring contact with transmitting antennas and their power source, diathermy equipment (found in hospitals), power transmission lines, radiation, and electrical equipment (i.e., that used for welding).

22. Is a cure going to be available soon?

Although we have made great strides in identifying the genes that cause HCM, a cure (such as with gene therapy) is still many years away because it represents an extremely complex and challenging scientific problem.

23. Should I consult with an HCM specialist? How do you know if someone is an HCM specialist?

The HCMA recommends that patients with HCM consult with a specialist in the field of HCM. This often involves some travel because there are relatively few such physicians who have focused their professional energy on this disease. Although it is not always convenient, traveling the distance to an HCM specialist or experienced center, has made a tremendous difference in the quality of life of many of our members. It is important to continue to work with your local cardiologist, however, and to keep the lines of communication open between all parties. Depending on the precise situation, consultations with an HCM specialist may be necessary only periodically. The HCMA keeps a registry of all cardiologists who either have specialized training and/or have authored articles on HCM, and are well-respected by their peers in this area.

24. Can my child participate in physical education classes or competitive athletics?

Organized competitive sports, with the exception of golf and bowling, are usually discouraged. Participation in physical education (gym) classes will be dependent on your child's health and the school system's guidelines. If the child is capable of participating in basic activities the school doctor or nurse may work with the physical education department to tailor an individualized program. In some school systems, this is called adaptive physical education. You should be aware, however, that certain gym class sports activities may be intense and truly competitive in nature, e.g., the traditional 600-yard run for speed, and these events should be avoided.

25. Can I scuba dive?

There is no information available that would suggest that scuba diving itself creates physiological alterations that are dangerous to HCM patients. However, diving requires submersion with a partner, and therefore any impairment in consciousness, incapacitation, or onset of symptoms (due to HCM) would also unavoidably impact the safety of another person. For these reasons, this particular sporting activity is probably not advisable for patients with HCM.

26. I have thought about taking Viagra. Are there any risks specifically for HCM patients?

Probably. Due to its known pharmacological actions, it is assumed that Viagra could occasionally have adverse consequences in anyone with HCM, and probably should be avoided.

27. I have been referred to a research center to be evaluated. What should I ask before I agree to participate?

Research is absolutely critical to all patients with HCM. It is the only way new information can be generated. Without novel research and new insights into the diagnosis, natural history, and treatment of HCM, our level of knowledge will not evolve and concepts of the disease will stagnate. However, it is also essential that you are very clear concerning the objectives of the researcher, center, and protocol that you are considering. You should know the benefits that you may receive, the risks that may be posed, the other treatment options or testing that is available, and the origin of the research funding. You should always ask for a written copy of the protocol and you should understand it completely before signing a consent form. You may also want to be aware of who may have access to your medical records and if the results of the testing are confidential. You should keep copies of all documentation you receive. While there are many superb HCM researchers throughout the world, do not assume that the person or center you are considering is the best for you (or even reputable) just because the institution may have a prominent name.

Glossary

This section provides a list of scientific terms commonly used with regard to HCM, defined in a relatively straightforward fashion, but avoiding medical jargon as much as possible. Some of these terms are also defined in the text, and are repeated here for completeness.

Ambulatory testing: Refers to tests performed while a person is performing his/her normal daily activities. (*See* Holter monitor.)

Angina: Chest pain or discomfort usually brought on by exertion and relieved by rest. Angina results from an insufficient oxygen supply to the heart muscle.

Angiography: An x-ray of the heart and blood vessels obtained at the time of cardiac catheterization with the injection of contrast dye. This test may be performed to assess the anatomy of the coronary arteries (blood vessels that supply the heart muscle).

Antibiotic prophylaxis: Administered prior to any dental procedures or surgical interventions for patients with the obstructive form of HCM, i.e., to prevent bacterial endocarditis and valve damage.

Anticoagulation: Treatment to reduce the potential of blood to form clots (e.g., with heparin or warfarin). Such treatment is used when there is a risk of clot formation in the heart, i.e., in the atria associated with atrial fibrillation.

Aorta: The main blood vessel, which arises from the left ventricle and carries blood from the heart to the rest of the body.

Apex: The bottom portion of the heart; the tip of the left ventricle.

Arrhythmia: An abnormal rhythm or irregularity of the heartbeat. The heartbeat may either be too fast (*tachycardia*) or too slow (*bradycardia*). Arrhythmias may cause symptoms such as palpitation or light-headedness, but many have more serious consequences, including sudden death.

Asymmetric hypertrophy: The circumstance in which some parts of the heart wall are thicker than other parts.

Atria: The two filling chambers of the heart, one on the right side and one on the left side. Blood is collected in the atria while the ventricles are contracting. This blood is then released from the atria into the ventricles when they are ready to fill.

Atrial fibrillation: A common type of arrhythmia in which the atria lose their normal contraction pattern and the heart rhythm becomes irregular. Atrial fibrillation may be transient or persistent.

Autosomal: Type of inheritance that is not linked to gender.

Autosomal dominant inheritance: A disease that is transmitted to each consecutive generation and occurs in about 50% of the relatives in a given generation.

Cardiac arrest: When the heart ceases to have an effective rhythm and contraction, and death is imminent.

Cardiac catheterization: A special invasive test used in patients with many forms of heart disease, including selected patients with HCM. A fine tube (catheter) is passed from a blood vessel (in the arm or groin) into the heart, using x-ray guidance, and pressures within the heart chambers are measured. Heart structure and function can be assessed with this procedure.

Cardiomyopathy: Refers to any disease predominantly involving the heart muscle; *cardio* refers to the heart and *myopathy* describes an abnormality of the heart muscle.

Concentric hypertrophy: The circumstance in which the left ventricular wall is thickened uniformly, also referred to as symmetric hypertrophy. This is a rare pattern in HCM.

Congestive heart failure: A condition where weakness in the beating action of the heart causes fluid retention and symptoms of shortness of breath and fatigue on exercise. While this form of heart failure may occur in a few HCM patients with progressive disease, heart failure in HCM much more commonly occurs by a different mechanism related to the impaired relaxation and filling of the ventricles in diastole (and in the presence of normal beating action of the heart).

Coronary artery disease: The common condition in which the coronary arteries (which deliver blood to the heart muscle) are narrowed by the accumulation of fatty plaque. When clots form on these plaques a "heart attack" (myocardial infarction) may result.

Diastole: Relaxation phase of the heart cycle when the ventricles passively fill with blood.

Dilatation: Enlargement or dilation of a heart chamber

Diuretics: Drugs that increase the production of urine by the kidneys and decrease fluid retention.

Dyspnea: Difficult or labored breathing; shortness of breath.

Echocardiogram (commonly shortened to **echo**): Echocardiography is the single most important test in the assessment of HCM. This is a noninvasive ultrasound scan of the heart, which produces an image of the chambers, walls, and valves, and can be viewed as a real-time movie (and is recorded permanently on videotape). *Doppler ultrasound* is part of the echocardiographic examination and produces a color-coded image of blood flow within the heart, detects areas of turbulent flow, and accurately measures the degree of obstruction. The pattern of filling of the left ventricle can also be assessed.

Electrocardiogram (or ECG): A very common test for all forms of heart disease. Electrodes are placed on the chest, wrists, and ankles to record electrical signals from the heart. Unlike the echocardiogram, the ECG does not produce a structural image of heart structure.

Electrophysiological study (or EPS): With this specialized test, catheters are introduced into the heart during cardiac catheterization. These catheters can both record and stimulate the electrical activity of the heart.

Endocarditis: An infection of the heart (usually of the valves) which may occur in HCM, although very rarely. Bacteria in the bloodstream can adhere to the internal surface of the heart or abnormal heart structures, particularly the mitral valve in HCM, and cause an infection.

Exercise stress testing: Exercise capacity may be tested using either a treadmill or a stationary bicycle. During an exercise test, a physician and technician monitor the patient's performance as well as symptoms, ECG, and blood pressure; sometimes the consumption of oxygen is also measured.

Genes and chromosomes: Genes are the code or blueprint that build all the tissues in the body. Each individual has thousands of genes and they are all present in every cell of the body. Genes come in pairs, one inherited from the mother and the other from the father. In each cell, the genes are grouped together by tiny, thread-like structures called chromosomes. Each person has 23 pairs of chromosomes.

Heart attack: Not appropriate terminology to describe a sudden collapse in HCM, but it is common terminology for an acute myocardial infarction due to coronary artery disease.

Heart block: Occasionally, the normal electrical signal cannot travel into the ventricles due to a pathologic disruption in the conducting system and a slow heart rate results. This situation can be identified by an ECG and corrected with a pacemaker.

Hypertrophic obstructive cardiomyopathy (HOCM): Commonly used term for HCM in the United Kingdom. However, this term implies that the disease is characterized by stenosis and outflow obstruction, which is not always the case.

Holter monitor: A continuous recording of the heartbeat over a 24- to 48-hour period. Adhesive electrodes are placed on the chest, with wires that connect to a special cassette recorder that is worn on a belt. A Holter monitor detects irregularity of the heartbeat, otherwise known as arrhythmia.

Hypertrophy: Literally means an increase in the muscle mass (or weight) of the heart. In HCM, hypertrophy refers specifically to an excessive thickening of the left ventricular wall.

Idiopathic hypertrophic subaortic stenosis (IHSS): An older name for HCM, used primarily in the U.S. in the 1960s. This term implies that the disease is always characterized by stenosis (i.e., outflow obstruction), which is erroneous.

Implantable cardioverter-defibrillator (ICD): A specialized and sophisticated device that is permanently implanted in the patient. It senses when the heart rate is excessively fast (which may represent a potentially lethal arrhythmia) and responds by either delivering a low-energy electrical shock or pacing the heart to restore the normal heart rhythm. An ICD can also serve as a pacemaker to pace the heart when the heart rate is too slow. Nevertheless, the ICD should not be confused with the conventional pacemaker. These are very different instruments with different objectives.

Mitral regurgitation: Refers to blood leaking back through the mitral valve during ejection. This occurs very commonly in HCM when there is outflow tract obstruction.

Murmur: Caused by turbulent blood flow within the heart. In HCM, the murmur is usually due to outflow obstruction, and the turbulence is produced by systolic anterior motion of the mitral valve or the associated mitral regurgitation. Not all murmurs, however, are of significance in patients with HCM and the doctor may regard the murmur as "innocent" and unrelated to the disease.

Mutation: A genetic defect that causes a change in the normal DNA code.

Myectomy (or myotomy-myectomy): An operation which may be performed in severely symptomatic patients with the obstructive form of HCM to remove a portion of the thickened muscle from the upper portion of the ventricular septum, and thereby relieve the outflow tract obstruction. This procedure is usually associated with long-lasting improvement of symptoms.

Myocardial disarray: When heart tissue from patients with HCM is viewed under a microscope, the normal parallel alignment of the muscle cells (myocytes) is usually absent. Instead, these cells (or bundles of cells) appear disorganized or in disarray, i.e., arranged at perpendicular and oblique angles to each other. There is no clinical test that can specifically detect disarray.

Myocardium: The specialized muscle that makes up the walls of the heart. It is this part of the heart that is the most abnormal in HCM.

Myosin: A protein within muscle cells that is prominently involved in normal contraction. In HCM, the gene that is responsible for coding myosin is abnormal and accounts for the disease in some families.

Noninvasive: Refers to tests that generally do not invade the integrity of the body, such as echocardiography or electrocardiography. (Cardiac catheterization, on the other hand, in which catheters are introduced through blood vessels into the heart, is an example of an invasive test.)

Outflow tract: The short channel in the heart through which blood ultimately passes from the ventricle into the aorta. It is essentially the upper portion of the left ventricle.

Outflow obstruction: Produced by the contact between mitral valve and thickened septum. This results in a pressure *gradient* between the upper and lower portions of the left ventricular cavity. Therefore, the terms *gradient* and *obstruction* are used synonymously.

Pacemaker: When the normal electrical impulse fails to be transmitted to the ventricles a pacemaker can be implanted to correct this problem. This involves inserting a small box containing a battery under the skin in the chest area, connected to fine wires which are inserted into a vein and to the heart, in order to deliver the necessary impulses.

Palpitation: An uncomfortable awareness of the heartbeat or rhythm. Palpitations may be due to normal heartbeats made more prominent by anxiety or exercise, or may in fact be caused by an arrhythmia. The presence of palpitations does not necessarily convey any prognostic significance in HCM, although on occasion (particularly when prolonged) they may be important signs about which you should advise your doctor.

Phenotype: The expression of a single gene (as in HCM), such as the thickened heart visualized by echocardiography.

Placebo: An interactive substance or preparation used in controlled experimental studies to determine the efficacy of medicinal substances. The placebo has no intrinsic therapeutic value but may induce psychological (or physiological) effects in patients that mimic "true" therapeutic results.

Recessive: An inherited trait that appears in only a single generation (usually in 1 in 4 individuals), i.e., is not evident in either the parents or children of the affected.

Sarcomere: The contractile unit of heart cells (myocytes).

Septum (ventricular septum): That portion of the heart wall that divides the right and left ventricles. In HCM, muscle thickening is usually most marked and most common in the septum. This observation has led to the descriptive term, *asymmetric septal hypertrophy*.

Syncope: Loss of consciousness by fainting.

Systole: The phase of heart cycle when blood is forcibly ejected from the ventricles, i.e., blood in the left ventricle flows into the aorta and to the major arteries and organs of the body.

Systolic anterior motion of the mitral valve (SAM): In some patients with HCM, the mitral valve moves forward and touches the septum (there should normally be a considerable gap between these structures) during the ejection of blood from the heart, thereby partially blocking the flow of blood from the outflow tract into the aorta. In the vast majority of patients, SAM is the mechanism of obstruction in HCM.

Ventricles: The two main (lower) pumping chambers of the heart; the right and left ventricles pump blood to the lungs and aorta, respectively. The left ventricle is that portion of the heart most commonly and predominantly affected in HCM.

Ventricular tachycardia: A type of arrhythmia in which repetitive and rapid premature beats arise within the ventricles.

Suggested References

1. Maron BJ. Hypertrophic cardiomyopathy. Lancet 1997;350: 127-133.
2. Spirito P, Seidman CE, McKenna WJ, Maron BJ. The management of hypertrophic cardiomyopathy. N Engl J Med 1997;336:775-785.
3. Wigle ED, Sasson Z, Henderson MA, et al. Hypertrophic cardiomyopathy: The importance of the site and the extent of hypertrophy. A review. Prog Cardiovasc Dis 1985;28:1-83.
4. Maron BJ, Mitchell JH. 26th Bethesda Conference. Recommendations for determining eligibility for competition in athletes with cardiovascular abnormalities. J Am Coll Cardiol 1994;24:845-899.
5. Maron BJ, Thompson PD, Puffer JC, et al. Cardiovascular preparticipation screening of competitive athletes. Circulation 1996;94: 850-856.
6. Wigle ED, Rakowski H, Kimball BP, Williams WG. Hypertrophic cardiomyopathy: Clinical spectrum and treatment. Circulation 1995;92:1680-1692.
7. Maron BJ. Hypertrophic cardiomyopathy. In Fuster V, Roberts R, Alexander RW, et al. (eds): Hurst's The Heart, 10th Edition. McGraw-Hill, New York, NY. In press.
8. McKenna WJ, Elliott PM. Hypertrophic cardiomyopathy. In Topol EJ (ed): Comprehensive Cardiovascular Medicine. Lippincott-Raven Publishers, Philadelphia, PA, pp 775-798.
9. Heric B, Lytle BW, Miller DP, et al. Surgical management of hypertrophic obstructive cardiomyopathy: Early and late results. J Thorac Cardiovasc Surg 1995;110:195-208.
10. Maron BJ, Shen W-K, Link MS, et al. Efficacy of implantable cardioverter-defibrillators for the prevention of sudden death in patients with hypertrophic cardiomyopathy. N Engl J Med 2000; 342:365-373.
11. Maron BJ, Olivotto I, Spirito P, et al. Epidemiology of hypertrophic cardiomyopathy-related death: Revisited in a large non-referral based patient population. Circulation 2000;102:858-864.
12. Spirito P, Bellone P, Harris KM, et al. Magnitude of left ventricular hypertrophy predicts the risk of sudden death in hypertrophic cardiomyopathy. N Engl J Med 2000;342:1778-1785.
13. Maron BJ, Moller JH, Seidman CE, et al. Impact of laboratory molecular diagnosis on contemporary diagnostic criteria for genetically transmitted cardiovascular diseases: Hypertrophic cardiomyopathy, long-QT syndrome, and Marfan syndrome. Circulation 1998;98:1460-1471.

14. Maron BJ, Casey SA, Poliac LC, et al. Clinical course of hypertrophic cardiomyopathy in a regional United States cohort. JAMA 1999;281:650-655.

15. Cecchi F, Olivotto I, Montereggi A, et al. Hypertrophic cardiomyopathy in Tuscany: Clinical course and outcome in an unselected regional population. J Am Coll Cardiol 1995;26:1529-1536.

16. Maron BJ, Nishimura RA, McKenna WJ, et al. Assessment of permanent dual-chamber pacing as a treatment for drug-refractory symptomatic patients with obstructive hypertrophic cardiomyopathy: A randomized, double-blind cross-over study (M-PATHY). Circulation 1999;99:2927-2933.

17. McCully RB, Nishimura RA, Tajik AJ, et al. Extent of clinical improvement after surgical treatment of hypertrophic obstructive cardiomyopathy. Circulation 1996;94:467-471.

18. Nishimura RA, Trusty JM, Hayes DL, et al. Dual-chamber pacing for hypertrophic cardiomyopathy: A randomized, double-blind cross-over study. J Am Coll Cardiol 1997;29:435-441.

19. Spirito P, Chiarella F, Carratino L, et al. Clinical course and prognosis of hypertrophic cardiomyopathy in an outpatient population. N Engl J Med 1989;320:749-755.

20. Maron BJ. Role of alcohol septal ablation in treatment of obstructive hypertrophic cardiomyopathy. Lancet 2000;355:425-426.

21. Spirito P, Rapezzi C, Bellone P, et al. Infective endocarditis in hypertrophic cardiomyopathy: Prevalence, incidence and indications for antibiotic prophylaxis. Circulation 1999;99:2132-2137.

22. Theodoro DA, Danielson GK, Feldt RH, et al. Hypertrophic cardiomyopathy in pediatric patients: Results of surgical treatment. J Thorac Cardiovasc Surg 1996;112:1589-1599.

23. Seggewiss H, Gleichman U, Faber L, et al. Percutaneous transluminal septal myocardial ablation in hypertrophic obstructive cardiomyopathy: Acute results and 3-month follow-up in 25 patients. J Am Coll Cardiol 1998;31:252-258.

24. Schwartz K, Carrier L, Guicheney P, Komajda M. Molecular basis of familial cardiomyopathies. Circulation 1995;91:532-540.

25. Marian AJ, Roberts R. Recent advances in the molecular genetics of hypertrophic cardiomyopathy. Circulation 1995;92:1336-1347.

26. Niimura H, Bachinski LL, Sangwatoraj S, et al. Mutations in the gene for human cardiac myosin-binding protein C and late-onset familial hypertrophic cardiomyopathy. N Engl J Med 1998;338:1248-1257.

27. Elliott PM, Poloniecki J, Dickie S, et al. Sudden death in hypertrophic cardiomyopathy: identification of high risk patient. J Am Coll Cardiol 2000;36:2212-2218.

HYPERTROPHIC CARDIOMYOPATHY ASSOCIATION

Membership Application

If you would like to become a member of the association, which will entitle you to receive copies of regular newsletters, benefit from a local contact network, and access advice and counseling, please complete and return this form.

If you do not wish to join, but feel that you can help us by making a contribution, please send your donation to the address below.

Please check the appropriate box.

☐ I would like to become a member of the association and I enclose $25.00 to cover the annual subscription fee, renewable annually, by September 1.

☐ Please check this box if you do not wish your name and telephone number to be given to other members.

☐ I enclose a donation to the Hypertrophic Cardiomyopathy Association for the amount of _____.

Checks should be made payable to HCMA and returned with this form to:

> HCMA
> PO Box 306
> Hibernia, NJ 07842
> Attn: Membership
>
> Tel: 973/983-7429 or
> Toll free: 877/329-4262
> Fax: 973/983-7489
> E-mail: *support@hcma-heart.com*

MR/MRS/MISS (Circle as appropriate)

Last name _____ First name _____

Address _____

_____

City/State _____ Zip code _____

Date of birth _____

Home tel. _____ Work tel. _____